Advancing Health in Developing Countries

ADVANCING HEALTH IN DEVELOPING COUNTRIES

The Role of Social Research

Edited by Lincoln C. Chen,
Arthur Kleinman, and Norma C. Ware

Prepared under the auspices of the Health Transition Project,
Center for Population Studies, Harvard University

AUBURN HOUSE
New York • Westport, Connecticut • London

Library of Congress Cataloging-in-Publication Data

Advancing health in developing countries : the role of social research
/ edited by Lincoln C. Chen, Arthur Kleinman, and Norma C. Ware.
  p.   cm.
Based on a workshop held at Harvard University in June 1989.
"Prepared under the auspices of the Health Transition Project,
Center for Population Studies, Harvard University."
Includes index.
ISBN 0–86569–034–0 (alk. paper)
1. Social medicine—Developing countries—Congresses.   I. Chen,
Lincoln C.   II. Kleinman, Arthur.   III. Ware, Norma C.   IV. Harvard
School of Public Health. Health Transition Project.
[DNLM: 1. Developing Countries—congresses.   2. Health Behavior—
congresses.   3. Health Promotion—trends—congresses.
4. Preventive Medicine—trends—congresses.   5. Social Change—
congresses.   WA 108 A244 1989]
RA418.A52   1992
362.1'09172'4—dc20
DNLM/DLC
for Library of Congress   91–26133

British Library Cataloguing in Publication Data is available.

Copyright © 1992 by Health Transition Project,
Center for Population Studies, Harvard University

Library of Congress Catalog Card Number: 91–26133
ISBN: 0–86569–034–0

First published in 1992

Auburn House, 88 Post Road West, Westport, CT 06881
An imprint of Greenwood Publishing Group, Inc.

Printed in the United States of America

The paper used in this book complies with the
Permanent Paper Standard issued by the National
Information Standards Organization (Z39.48–1984).

P

In order to keep this title in print and available to the academic community, this edition
was produced using digital reprint technology in a relatively short print run. This would
not have been attainable using traditional methods. Although the cover has been changed
from its original appearance, the text remains the same and all materials and methods
used still conform to the highest book-making standards.

Contents

Preface

Among the great achievements of humankind in the twentieth century have been the enormous improvements in health worldwide. The pace and character of these health gains, however, exhibit marked variability between nations and communities, reflecting global disparities in human achievement. Despite these inequities, the overall pattern has been truly remarkable. Few would have predicted at the beginning of this century that average life spans would be approaching 80 years in many economically advanced societies and that the gap between developing and industrialized countries would be narrowing as we approach the close of the century.

What has accounted for these phenomenal achievements? Many theories have been advanced—from the marvels of modern medical technology to fundamental social and economic developments that have provided adequate food, shelter, clothing, and effective health care. A common basis for these advances is the enormous explosion of knowledge enabling humankind to better control the environment. This knowledge, generated by a human process called research, has provided the underlying basis of technology development and socioeconomic growth that have fueled the acceleration of health improvement.

Although it is a virtual certainty that the production of knowledge has enabled humankind to better control the environment and reduce the threat of unnecessary illness and premature death, the mechanisms through which health research links to effective health action are, at best, incompletely understood. In the natural and life sciences, the accepted paradigm is of laboratory developments leading to technologies for field applications that are then disseminated through mass-scale so-

cial systems, such as health care systems or commercial business enter-
prises. For the social and behavioral sciences, few paradigms explain
how social research translates into more effective social action.
Some have argued that social research helps to identify the nature of
health problems, thereby improving the targeting of social interventions.
Others have hypothesized that research can help guide social interventions in the more effective application of available technology and tools.
Still others have proposed that the impact of knowledge is through
changing mass attitudes and behavior, profoundly affecting individual
behavior and community norms surrounding health processes. Examples abound with regard to these propositions. Epidemiologic and social
research provides information on the magnitude, distribution, and
changing trends of particular health problems. Operational or evaluative
research can contribute to improved efficiency and effectiveness of health
care delivery systems. Surveys of knowledge, attitude, and practice
(KAPs) can generate insights on how educational messages can be formulated and directed to influence health-related behavior. But, despite
this plethora of specific illustrations of research-to-action linkages, there
have been few overarching theories to guide our understanding of how
social research realizes its payoff in terms of social action for health.

The chapters in this book attempt to address this basic question. The
book represents the products of an extremely rich set of papers presented
at a workshop organized by the Harvard Center for Population and
Development Studies and conducted at the American Academy of Arts
and Sciences in Cambridge, Massachusetts in June 1989. Supported by
a generous grant from the Rockefeller Foundation, workshop participants attempted to address how health action could be influenced by
social research. The organizing theme of the workshop was the "health
transitions," a concept of the social nature of changing health status in
human populations. The underlying premise of the workshop was that
research to elucidate the dynamic determinants and consequences of
health transitions would help guide health interventions.

The workshop papers and commentaries are organized into three parts
in this book. Following an introductory chapter by Sally Findley, then
program officer at the Rockefeller Foundation responsible for health
transition activities, the first part contains three chapters on social, behavioral, and anthropological research and its relevance to health and
social change. The second part contains five case studies of the linkages
between social research and action. The case studies were carefully selected to represent key health problems linked directly to remedial action. Two of the health problems are global in scope (smoking and AIDS)
and two are of very high priority to many developing countries (malaria
and diarrhea). The final part contains two chapters addressing direct
linkages between social research and social interventions. The first of

these examines research linkages to economic policy, while the second proposes modifications in the process of research to improve its translation into action. The final chapter summarizes the workshop deliberations and proposes new ways of thinking about the relationship.

The editors are grateful to many who made the workshop and this volume possible. Grant support from the Rockefeller Foundation for the workshop and this publication is gratefully acknowledged. We are particularly indebted to Ms. Ellen Hopkins, Ms. Colleen Murphy, and other staff at the Harvard Center for Population and Development Studies who managed the complex logistics associated with the workshop. Dr. Norma Ware, one of the editors, devoted considerable time and energy to communicating with contributors and editing for publication the chapters in this volume. We, the editors, assume responsibility for the shortcomings.

Advancing Health in Developing Countries

Introduction: Addressing the Health Transition Research Agenda—Can We Connect Findings with Action?

SALLY E. FINDLEY

The twentieth century has witnessed remarkable changes in health patterns worldwide. In industrialized nations, childhood mortality has dropped nearly thirtyfold to around 10 per 1,000. Similar decreases have recently taken place in some parts of the developing world, while in other nations infant mortality rates have plateaued at 100 to 150 per 1,000 live births. Differential provision of effective preventive and curative medical services may contribute in part to the variation in the pace of mortality decline. Some scientists, however, attribute this variation to differences in social, economic, and political factors, such as levels of female education and autonomy, nutritional adequacy, and political priorities for health (Caldwell and Caldwell 1985; Halstead, Walsh, and Warren 1985). It is becoming increasingly evident that further reductions in mortality will require greater complementarity between social changes and direct health service inputs. If specific mechanisms of social and behavioral changes were understood, it would be possible to better design health and developmental interventions to accelerate health improvements without having to wait for fulfillment of the elusive goals of universal education or socioeconomic development.

A "health transition" concept has been adopted by many to guide thinking about the social transformations that accelerate the process of achieving health for all. In recognition of the mounting evidence that biomedical technology alone cannot produce further dramatic declines in mortality, the Rockefeller Foundation sponsored three internal workshops in 1989 to discuss the health transition concept and to determine, based on the evidence, whether it would be possible to launch new research initiatives that could provide developing countries with information needed for accelerating their social and health transformations. The first workshop was held in May 1989 at the Australian National University in Canberra, Australia. The meeting focused on the concept of the health transition and existing evidence regarding the social, behavioral, and cultural determinants of health change. The presentations underscored the dynamic and complex nature of the health transitions. Workshop participants agreed that sociocultural norms, household economics, and community development are critical components of the transition process.

The second workshop, held in June 1989 at the London School of Hygiene and Tropical Medicine, considered methodologies for measuring health transition processes. Participants concluded that in general, existing research methodologies were adequate for the study of the health transition. These methods, however, needed to be combined in new ways—by mixing methodologies and disciplines, combining quantitative and qualitative methods, adopting multidisease perspectives, and developing multilevel studies in which family and community levels could be integrated.

Theoretical knowledge of the processes that might facilitate a more rapid improvement in health is not sufficient. Knowing how social changes can be produced is not the same as implementing the programs that incorporate these principles. For many reasons, social science research often fails to guide social policy in the ways researchers hope (Nathan 1988; Rule 1978). Not only must research identify specific mechanisms of change, it must do so through a process that opens those findings to potential users, whether they are health planners, program managers, community development agents, or others whose activities touch on pertinent action.

The research process and its relation to action was the subject of the third health transition workshop, held at Harvard University in June 1989. Participants were asked to analyze case studies describing actual research projects and their policy and programmatic sequelae. Discussions then focused on those aspects of the research process that may have been conducive to successful application.

This book is an outgrowth of the Harvard workshop. The first set of chapters outlines social scientists' views of the issues involved in conceptualizing the behavioral changes implicated in the health transition. The second set of chapters presents case studies that illustrate the process of actually applying social science on behalf of efforts to alter health behaviors. The book closes with three chapters that address the question of what social science research can contribute to the improvement of health.

As a background to these discussions, this chapter reviews the health transition concepts, identifies topics for future research, and summarizes the major points made in the chapters. This introduction concentrates on outlining a number of considerations likely to affect the application of health transition research—issues that are considered in much greater depth in the remainder of the volume.

TOWARD A DEFINITION OF THE HEALTH TRANSITION

To refer to the broad social factors underlying systematic changes in health status of human populations, John Caldwell has recently coined the term "health transition." The health transition concept encompasses those changes in social norms, social structure, and individual behavior that result in better health (Caldwell 1990). Although the health transition is reflected in the mortality and epidemiological transitions, its focus is not mortality per se, but rather the social processes through which a society improves its health and life expectancy.

Consistent with the emphasis on the social determinants of health, the health transition defines health as more than the absence of disease. Health is construed as the ability to function. The best approximation of this definition of health was suggested by Dubos, who defined health as a "physical and mental state fairly free of discomfort and pain which permits persons to function effectively and as long as possible in the environment" (1965:351).

The social dimensions most relevant to the health transition are the perception of and the ability to control one's environment and daily life so that health is maintained. Societies in early stages of the health transition tend to enforce long-standing social controls that prescribe certain behaviors for dealing with illness and maintaining health. As the transition progresses, social and community structures change to incorporate additional health-seeking and health-maintenance behaviors. This social transformation is the key to the health transition process.

In theory, the health transition typifies the social and behavioral changes involved when good health comes within reach of the broad masses of a given population. This does not mean that illness or sickness is eliminated; it does mean, however, that a community has available a broader and more effective range of mechanisms through which to prevent and treat disease. Some of these, such as vaccinations, are explicitly targeted against specific diseases. Others, such as clean water or enhanced educational opportunities for women, are interventions that affect health status indirectly. In addition to these community supports for good health, changes in social norms and in behavioral patterns enable people to avoid serious diseases for much of their childhood and adulthood. Together, these factors produce changes in attitudes and in the way people respond to disease and the threat of ill health. These changes, in turn, modify the incidence and prevalence of disease.

Changes in the configuration of disease during the course of the health transition have been well described by researchers concerned with the epidemiological transition (see, for example, Omran 1971). These changes may be grouped into three stages.

The first stage is characterized by a high level of infectious and parasitic diseases. In the context of malnutrition and generally poor health, children experience high mortality risks; hence, life expectancy is brief and high mortality and high morbidity coexist. The total disease burden is high (Ghana Health Assessment Project Team 1981; Manton, Dowd, and Woodbury 1986; Walsh 1985).

In the second stage, the major infectious epidemics are substantially reduced. Mortality begins to fall, but morbidity may not yet decline proportionately. In today's transitional countries, even as water and airborne infectious diseases are decreasing, reductions in morbidity are retarded by the continuing prevalence of tropical diseases. Eight such parasitic diseases are particularly problematic. They are: malaria, onchocerciasis, schistosomiasis, tuberculosis, leprosy, polio, leishmaniasis, and filariasis (Walsh 1985). All except one of these chronic diseases are progressively disabling. Their effects are hardly perceptible immediately after infection, but as years go by without treatment, impairment steadily increases, sometimes leading to almost complete disability. This is the progression, for example, in onchocerciasis, otherwise known as river blindness.

In the later stages of the transition, water and airborne infectious and parasitic diseases have a much lower incidence. These are replaced, however, by higher rates of chronic, degenerative, or accident-related diseases (Ruzicka and Kane 1990). Because many of these diseases have low incidence rates among young children, the childhood years tend to be more disease free. Levels of illness in the population rise with age, however, due both to accidents and to diseases related to the man-made environment or to aging. Recent evidence from China, other parts of Asia, and Mexico shows that today's late transitional societies have high levels of cardiovascular disease and malignant neoplasms. Both of these are considered to be diseases that emerge from the transition (Feachem 1990; Frenk, Bobadilla, Sepulvida, and Cervanto 1989; Reddy 1989).

During the transition, socioeconomic inequalities and regional developmental differences may result in marked heterogeneity in the tempo of health change. At any given time, some groups will be experiencing the disease and mortality patterns of the earlier stages, while others will be subject to later transitional diseases. In Mexico, for example, researchers have found marked regional differences in the epidemiological transition (Aspe and Beristáin 1989). Some populations may even exhibit signs of multiple stages simultaneously, as in the peripheral settlements of Sao Paulo or Bombay, where residents bear the disease burdens of both poverty and industrial pollution (Crook, Ramasubban, and Singh 1991). This pattern is widespread in India, which has greater prevalence of both acute respiratory inflections and degenerative diseases (Reddy 1989).

In light of this, it would be inaccurate to talk about the health transition in developing countries as if it were a synchronized change from high mortality and high morbidity to low mortality and low morbidity. Rather, the health transition should be viewed as a transition from diseases that are linked to natural infection processes to ones that are largely the consequence of the man-made environment. In an early transitional society, the population faces significant mortality risks early in life. In later transitional settings, the significant health problems emerge later, when the cumulative effects of aging or exposure to various pollutants manifest themselves (Alter and Riley 1989). In the intermediate stages, childhood morbidity due to infectious diseases may be lower, but childhood and adult morbidity related to parasitic or recurrent infectious diseases will continue to be high (Corbett 1989). Accelerating beyond or easing these transitional problems challenges us to look for innovative social mechanisms that reduce the risks of illness across the disease spectrum.

A HEALTH TRANSITION RESEARCH AGENDA

Much like the fertility transition, the health transition involves a broadly interactive set of changes in individual attitudes and behaviors, in family roles and resource allocation patterns, and in the nature of community supports for better health. Individuals and families play an important role in the protection and preservation of health, but community infrastructure and health care services define the range of resources and expectations available to individuals in fulfilling this task.

What are the driving forces for change in this interactive system? There are three distinctive perspectives on the levels and processes of change: sociocultural norms, household economics, and community development and institutions.

Sociocultural Norms

There is widespread agreement that we must understand more about the ways health-related behaviors are shaped by sociocultural norms. It is assumed that health attitudes and behaviors change during the transition, but we know very little about the forces driving such changes, or whether they can be accelerated through planned interventions.

Just as earlier researchers identified culture as a key factor in the fertility transition (Handwerker 1986), recent studies have shown how culture shapes people's ideas about the level of health they can reasonably expect to attain and the options they have for achieving that level (Foster 1984; Heggenhougen 1991; Janzen 1990; Kleinman 1980). Culture provides the system of meanings through which women and other primary care-givers define and deal with sickness. Culture also outlines the responsibilities of governments or communities with respect to the maintenance of public health (Cantrelle and Locoh 1990; Johansson 1990).

Promising areas for additional research on sociocultural influences on health behavior include the following:

The interplay between changes in attitudes and behaviors. Several studies suggest that health transitions have been linked to spreading perceptions that disease is not a normal state and that individuals can and should take steps to avoid illness (Dubos 1965; Kleinman 1980; Streatfield and Singarimbun 1986; Visaria 1990). When new health care technologies are introduced, those who believe that disease can be controlled are more likely to adopt them. But how do attitudes toward disease and health care change, and how do changes in attitudes facilitate changes in behavior? Can behavioral changes, that is, new health care technologies, be introduced in advance of attitudinal change?

Self-reliance. There is some evidence that attitudinal changes during the transition involve an increase in self-reliance or self-efficacy—the sense that each person, but especially women, can take charge of his or her life (Caldwell, Caldwell, Gajanayake, Orubuloye, Pieris, and Reddy 1990; Cosminsky 1990; Nag 1990; Nations and Farias 1990). A shift in the locus of control away from elders (or others) and toward the individual is also part of this process (Simons 1989).

But how does a greater sense of self-efficacy actually translate into better health? What are the mechanisms by which societies allow or facilitate changes in their expectations for individual autonomy and efficacy? Is maternal education one of them, as suggested by Cleland and van Ginneken (1988) and Caldwell, Caldwell, Gajanayake, Orubuloye, Pieris, and Reddy (1990)? What other factors shift the locus of control to individuals and to women specifically?

Perceptions of the etiology and treatment of disease. During the transition, perceptions that disease can be avoided and effectively treated become more widespread. The search for health leads many to combine traditional, allopathic, and even spiritual healing methods (Finerman 1990; Good 1987; Janzen 1978). There is less patience with treatment that does not work, and care-givers are quicker to turn to alternatives when initial attempts to cure the disease prove unsuccessful (Caldwell, Caldwell, Gajanayake, Orubuloye, Pieris, and Reddy 1990; Sushama 1990).

What social and behavioral changes are linked to the expansion of the care repertoire and increased demand for effective treatments? There is some evidence that female education is a catalyst in this process, but additional research is needed to identify other pathways of change.

Increased role of the state. During the transition there is a growing awareness of "public health" and the duty of the state to protect common health (Ewbank and Preston 1990; Van de Walle and Van de Walle 1990; Woods 1990). A central issue is the increasing understanding that poor sanitation and unsatisfactory hygiene contribute to the spread of disease. The concept that people have a right to medical care is also part of this new consciousness (Dubos 1965; Nag 1990).

In addition to the diffusion of information about processes of contagion and transmission, what social and economic factors promote the state's role in guarding public health and welfare? How important are political factors, such as the views of political parties and trade unions?

Household Economics

Even if attitudinal changes support improved health behaviors, poverty may make it difficult, if not impossible, for people to adopt these behaviors. Accordingly, the health transition research agenda also focuses on household economics. The issue here is the ability of families to "buy" good health.

Economic models assume that families want good health but that their ability to actually achieve it is constrained by (1) limited resources (low income, poor diet, poor housing), (2) inadequate information (e.g., no knowledge of practices or inputs that can efficiently increase health levels for household members), and (3) lack of access to modern technologies (e.g., primary health care services or public health measures) (Cebu Study Team 1991; DaVanzo and Gertler 1990; Schultz 1985). Aspects of community infrastructure and physical environment also affect a household's disease risk and, therefore, the level of effort needed to maintain health (Anker and Knowles 1980; DaVanzo and Gertler 1990; Mosley and Chen 1984; Schultz 1985).

Research reports from around the world attest to the fact that for the poor, lack of money and free time are major constraints on the achievement of good health (Cosminsky 1990; Rosenzweig and Schultz 1981; Strauss 1988; Visaria 1990;). Does this mean that we must wait for economic growth before widespread improvements in health can be expected?

Case studies of China, Sri Lanka, Kerala State in India, Costa Rica, and Cuba show that it is possible for societies to achieve better health despite the constraints of limited economic development (Halstead, Walsh, and Warren 1985). Even more intriguing are household-level studies showing that some families in impoverished settings are significantly more successful in improving the health of their members than other, equally poor households (Basu 1990; Cosminsky 1990; Das Gupta 1990; Tekca and Shorter 1984). More studies are needed to identify the mechanisms by which some poor people are able to achieve better health than others.

There is a virtual consensus in the research literature that maternal education is a key intervening variable influencing the production of good health, especially among young children (Basu 1990; Caldwell 1979; Carvajal and Burgess 1978; Farah and Preston 1982; Haines and Avery 1982; Rosenzweig and Schultz 1981; Strauss 1988; Ware 1984). However, the exact mechanisms by which maternal education affects health have not yet been identified. In their review of studies considering the relationship of maternal education to health, Cleland and van Ginneken (1988) find the most promising explanation in the proposition that educated mothers make more use of health services. The identification of alternative explanations will require comparison of cases in which maternal education does and does not have a strong impact upon health status.

Priority research questions on household health production strategies center on the following themes:

Acquisition of information about health care technologies. How do households learn of improved techniques? How does low income constrain the acquisition of improved care technologies? How does education speed the uptake of improved health care techniques?

Resources to purchase health care. Which health inputs are most cost effective for a family to purchase? What limits use of these inputs? Which types of households are more likely to allocate marginal increases in income to health?

Health care decisionmaking. When there are conflicts over the allocation of household resources to health, how are they resolved? Which decision-making patterns increase either the level of the efficiency of household health production? Where does the autonomy of women fit into the economic model?

The effect of women's education. What are the mechanisms through which increases in the level of women's education result in improved health?

Community Development and Institutions

The health transition concept highlights the role of community socioeconomic changes in accelerating a society-wide transition toward better health. Indeed, a major hypothesis in health transition research is that economic development leads to better health only insofar as development changes trigger community-level changes in attitudes and behavior that permit widespread acquisition of good health. Which community characteristics affect the translation of economic growth into better health? The following have been identified as priority areas of research:

Availability and distribution of food and shelter. The inverse relation between economic development and individual mortality has been shown to depend on income distribution, availability and price of food, and average living standards (Lipton and deKadt 1988; Longhurst 1984; Martorell and Sharma 1985; Millard, Ferguson, and Khaila 1990; Rodgers 1979). Detailed studies are needed to understand how seasonal and chronic food shortages affect health behaviors, not just dietary intake or body weight. These studies could suggest ways in which food and agricultural development programs could be modified to better protect families' health in case of food shortfall.

Environmental sanitation. Studies have shown that clean water supplies, waste disposal systems, and disease vector control programs affect mortality levels independent of the aggregate income effect (Briscoe 1984; Dubos 1965; Bradley, Garelick, and Mata 1983; Grosse 1980). Some argue that provision of infrastructure and sanitation services should be the first step in promoting a health transition (Dubos 1965).

But in some cases wells or improved sanitation have not been associated with improved health (Basu 1990; Feachem 1985; Rosenfield 1990). What are the conditions under which clean water supplies and sanitation systems correlate with improved health? Where water and sanitation systems are inadequate, what household behaviors or community practices (e.g., livestock stabling, laundry locations) might offset the deleterious effects of poor sanitation or inadequate water supplies?

Availability and quality of health care services. The relationship between health care services and health status has been a subject of debate ever since it was demonstrated that a decline in disease prevalence can precede significant innovations in medical care (Dubos 1961; McKeown 1976). Correlation analyses continue to show only weak bivariate relations between measures of the supply of health services and actual health (Alachakar and Serow 1988; Grosse 1980).

However, micro-level case studies often show the availability and use of primary health care services have been instrumental in reductions in mortality (Halstead, Walsh, and Warren 1985; Hardiman 1986; Morley, Rohde, and Williams 1983). In Kerala, for example, the transition was expedited by the provision of simple curative health facilities within walking distance of the entire urban and rural population (Panikar and Soman 1984). In Mlomp, Senegal, the most important community factor associated with declining child mortality rates was the extension of health care services and an effective outreach program that encouraged their use (Pison, Lefebre, Enel, and Trape 1989).

How do levels of economic development, community infrastructure, attitudes toward women, and organization of economic activities affect the uptake of primary health care services? What health service characteristics increase the positive effect of the facilities on community health levels? Answers to these questions can help health planners tailor services to communities at various stages of the health transition.

CONNECTING FINDINGS WITH ACTION

How can research on this agenda serve the goal of actually accelerating the health transition? This is the general question addressed by the chapters in this volume.

Appropriate Models of Behavioral Change

If the litmus test of social science research is the degree to which it actually guides the implementation of programs that successfully change health-related behaviors, it is essential that appropriate models of behavioral change be used. The chapters in the first section of the volume are concerned with how health-relevant changes in attitudes and behaviors are best conceptualized.

The contribution of anthropological approaches to the development of models of behavioral change is the subject of the chapter by Ware, Christakis and Kleinman. These authors argue that any adequate conceptualization of the health transition must explicitly incorporate the effects of micro-level social processes, as well as large-scale socioeconomic and political changes. A review of the cross-cultural literature on illness behavior—the response of an individual to somatic changes perceived as symptoms—provides the empirical foundation for the argument.

Anthropological studies of illness behavior reveal wide cultural variation in the ways symptoms are defined, causes of illness are construed, and diagnoses and treatment are sought. Traditional healing and biomedicine are combined, for example, in a number of different ways in situations of medical pluralism around the world.

The clear implication of the anthropological evidence is that unless the significance of local-level cultural variation is incorporated into theoretical models of behavior change, our understanding of the dynamics of the health transition will remain partial at best.

In a similar vein, the chapter by Weiss emphasizes the need for theoretical models of behavioral change that take a range of different considerations into account. Personal, familial, social, and environmental factors that impede individual attempts to modify their behavior must be represented in any adequate theory we develop. For social science research to be useful to policymakers, we must question models of behavioral change that assume a high degree of self-responsibility, initiative, and self-regulation. Rather, the belief systems and behavioral incentives that structure and shape everyday life must be integrated into our theoretical framework. Such integrated models will help us to understand why relatively simple behavioral changes that could do so much to improve health are not adopted.

The role of extrapersonal factors in influencing behavioral modifications is also stressed in Mechanic's chapter. He focuses particularly on underlying societal values that may predispose individuals to adopt new behaviors. Given that health is heavily influenced by daily living patterns, it is more likely to be affected by social norms than by conscious, explicit health behaviors at the individual level. Mechanic argues for greater attention to various environmental mechanisms that might induce behavioral change, with or without prior change in underlying attitudes. He challenges us to consider how such external inducements might interact with ongoing normative changes, such as those accelerated by education. He also recommends close study of processes associated with psychological modernity, a set of attitudes that fosters the adoption of innovative social roles and practices.

Mechanic concludes that our present models are insufficient to adequately show how specific interventions, such as education, shape attitudes and behavior. Studying the normative and extra-personal constraints on behavior modification may provide important clues about why people do not translate intentions for good health into appropriate behaviors. This information is critical to developing programs that foster health-promoting behavioral change.

Thus, the chapters constituting Part I all argue, in one way or another, for a conceptualization of health-related behavior change that moves beyond the level of the individual to incorporate a range of micro- and macro-level social influences. Part II of the volume turns from conceptual to empirical concerns.

Empirical Studies of Behavioral Change

The five chapters constituting Part II are case study examples of social science research on health-related behavioral change. They provide an overview of the various forms such change can take—historical or comparative analyses, intervention trials, program evaluation, the application of innovative methodologies. The cases were selected to represent health problems that are global (common to both industrialized and developing countries, such as smoking and AIDS) as well as those specific to the developing world (e.g., malaria and diarrhea). The case study chapters are accompanied by short commentaries. The major points of these five chapters are summarized in the following paragraph.

In his analysis of the decline of smoking in the United States, Brandt illustrates some of the complexities of inducing behavioral change. Before the late 1970s, there was no lack of scientific evidence pointing out the health risks of smoking. Nor were government or the media incapable of accurately communicating these risks. Nonetheless, the antismoking campaign faltered until there were fundamental transformations in the meaning of smoking. With the release of evidence regarding the risks of passive smoke inhalation, or sidestream smoking, individual smokers could no longer overlook the dangers their habit posed to others. While they might continue to believe in their right to ruin their own bodies (an expression of self-determination), their sense of collective responsibility required acquiescence to smoking regulations. Thus, changes in behavior were induced by a combination of regulatory acts and attitudinal changes. Brandt's analysis demonstrates the wide range of process variables—from personal to societal—that need to be considered if we are to launch successful campaigns of behavioral change.

Differences in the perceptions of, and the importance attached to, the AIDS epidemic in Great Britain, Sweden, and the United States are contrasted in Fox's chapter. He shows how these differences have significant implications for the formulation of relevant health policy. Fox uses this comparison of varying responses to the AIDS epidemic to illustrate the importance of understanding the particularities of policymaking in a given setting—"how and why a country sets the health policies it does"—in order to insure that social science research is not only relevant, but also meets the specific needs of those it is designed to serve. Social scientists maximize the likelihood that the results of their research will be implemented by developing an understanding of the policy-making process in the situation to which their work is directed, and then tailoring their efforts to fit the requirements that particular situation presents.

The analysis offered by Sawyer and Sawyer demonstrates how substantive findings from social science research can yield concrete program recommendations. In their case these are specific improvements in the Brazilian government's antimalarial campaign. After documentation the failures of the existing, technologically based mosquito control program, these authors go on to argue for the value of making the poor settlers of the Amazon region the target of future control efforts. In carrying out their research, Sawyer and Sawyer discovered that the settlers themselves had implemented efforts to control the mosquito population. On the basis of this finding, they recommend vector control programs designed to build upon already existing self-help efforts. The results of this research point to ways of coordinating government and local efforts to bring about health-enhancing behavioral change.

The intervention study of diarrheal disease management presented by Lopez de Romana and his colleagues illustrates Mechanic's point about the influence of extrapersonal factors on attitudinal transformation. In Peru, as in many developing countries, children often decrease their food intake during episodes of childhood diarrhea. Yet, research by these authors showed that children who received solid food throughout a diarrheal episode were better protected against weight loss. To encourage women to feed solid foods to their infants during episodes of diarrhea, they combined old and new technologies in an ingenious educational campaign. The central element of their strategy was to introduce a baby food that resembled a popular snack. Using radio, press, and demonstrations in women's clubs, they trained a significant number of women to prepare the food. Subsequent surveys showed that many mothers did in fact change their behavior in the desired direction as a result of the intervention.

The last case study, authored by Lanata and his colleagues, shows how social science methodologies developed for use in other settings can be adapted to address health-related research questions of direct relevance to policy decisions. These investigators applied a survey technique previously used for industrial quality control to the assessment of immunization coverage in the area in and around Lima, Peru. The "Lot Quality Assurance Sampling" method is a way of measuring conformity to a predetermined standard of "quality" in each of a set of designated units. In the Peruvian context, it was used to estimate the proportion of completed vaccinations in local health posts. Officials were able to use the data to make needed changes in implementation of the immunization campaign. The result was improved program performance and increased interest on the part of policymakers in making use of social science research.

Social Science Research and the Improvement of Health

From the consideration of conceptual issues in research on the health transition in Part I of the volume, to a focus on empirical case studies in Part II, we move finally to three chapters that directly address the fundamental question of what social science research can contribute to improved health.

Birdsall responds to this question by reviewing the current status of research on the relationship between health and economic development. Of particular interest is the fact that she discusses not only the effect of development on health, but also the impact of health on development. Birdsall concludes that good research can make a difference to health by influencing policy and program development. Research on the determinants of health at the household level are particularly important, for example, in helping to bring about health improvements that depend on behavioral change. Studies of the consequences, or "social returns," of investments in health in developing countries will be necessary to defend continued allocation of resources to health care.

In his chapter, Mosley challenges social scientists to integrate research with health planning and administration. If research maintains this kind of inclusive orientation, it will capture the interest of policymakers and will generate its own learning process. Then, when it is time to implement the research findings, those involved in a position to do so will be more receptive and ready to carry out recommendations.

To facilitate the type of organizational learning process, research must be more problem-oriented. The researcher must frame the research in concrete terms relevant to specific program or community situations. Whereas in standard scientific research the researcher starts with hypothesis formulation, in applied action research he or she starts by outlining a concrete problem. Specialized knowledge of social processes is then used to formulate a trial solution. As in experimental laboratory research, these trial solutions become the research hypotheses. The outcome of the research is not the elaboration of theory but decisions about how the solution works in particular settings (Boehm 1982).

Thus, Mosley's arguments parallel those of others who claim that social science researchers must carefully consider who their research will benefit and how, and then ensure that the research allows for the proper translation of results for these clients (Rule 1978). Researchers should ask policy and program officials what prevents them from taking effective action, and then they should design their studies to address the agenda defined by the problems policymakers confront (Nathan 1988).

The potential of social science research to contribute to improved health is addressed by Chen through a summary of the workshop proceedings in the volume's closing chapter. The summary is divided into four parts reflecting major themes that emerged from the workshop discussions. The first part reviews unresolved challenges, among them the following questions: Are the social sciences needed? How does social science make a difference in the everyday lives of people living in the community. The significance and usefulness of the health transition concept itself is addressed, and reaffirmed, in the second part. The third section recapitulates major conceptual points about the relation of social research to action, citing direct and indirect, or mediated, relations as two different possibilities. The summary ends with suggestions for guidelines to direct the implementation of a successful health transition program.

CONCLUSION

The health transition research agenda is complex. Some researchers will be focused on sociocultural influences on behavior, which calls for intensive micro-level studies of individuals, families, and communities. Others will grapple with the issues of resource allocation, looking at economic structures, household choices, and the production of good health. Still others will examine developmental and community-wide influences on both resource allocation patterns and health attitudes and behaviors. Coordination of these diverse elements of the overall process will call for regular communication between researchers and unrelenting attempts to make connections among research activities.

Focusing on why we are doing research and how we expect it to serve our larger ends will help us shape our studies to make the needed connections. All researchers must deal with the need to use theoretical models that help to identify processes of change and external contraints on change. These models will provide clues to guide implementation. Equally important is the tailoring of research to better integrate it with action concerns. In many different ways the contributors to this volume underscore the importance of a close partnership between researchers and implementors. By comparing the ways in which particular research projects address implementation issues, we will be better able to serve the purpose of applying the substantive research agenda on behalf of the health transition.

REFERENCES

Alachakar, A., and W. Serow. 1988. The Socioeconomic Determinants of Mortality: An International Comparison. *Genus* 44, 3–4 December.

Alter, G., and J. Riley. 1989. Frailty and Mortality in Historical Populations. *Population Studies* 43:1:25–45.

Anker, R., and J. C. Knowles. 1980. An Empirical Analysis of Mortality Differentials in Kenya at the Macro and Micro Levels. *Economic Development and Cultural Change*, October.

Aspe, Pedro, and Javier Beristáin. 1989. Distribución de los Servicios Educativos y de Salud. *Salud Publica de Mexico* 31 (2), Mar.–April, pp. 240–83.

Basu, A. 1990. Cultural Influences on Child Health in a Delhi Slum: In What Way Is Urban Poverty Preferable to Rural Poverty? In *What We Know about the Health Transition: The Proceedings of an International Workshop, Canberra, May 1989.* J. C. Caldwell, S. Findley, P. Caldwell, M. G. Santow, W. H. Cosford, J. Braid, and D. Broers-Freeman, eds. Canberra: Australian National University Press.

Boehm, V. 1982. Research in the "Real World": A Conceptual Model. In *Making It Happen: Designing Research with Implementation in Mind.* Innovations in

Methodology No. 3. D. M. Hakel, Melvin Sorcher, Michael Beer, and Joseph L. Moses, eds. Beverly Hills: Sage Publications.

Briscoe, J. 1984. Technology and Child Survival: The Example of Sanitary Engineering. *Population and Development Review* 10:237–53.

Caldwell, J. C. 1979. Education as a Factor in Mortality Decline: An Examination of Nigerian Data. *Population Studies* 33:395–415.

———. 1990. Introductory Thoughts on the Health Transition. In *What We Know about the Health Transition: The Proceedings of an International Workshop, Canberra, May 1989*. J. C. Caldwell, S. Findley, P. Caldwell, M. G. Santow, W. H. Cosford, J. Braid, and D. Broers-Freeman, eds. Canberra: Australian National University Press.

Caldwell, J. C., and P. Caldwell. 1985. Education and Literacy as Factors in Health. In *Good Health at Low Cost*. S. B. Halstead, J. Walsh, and K. Warren, eds. New York: Rockefeller Foundation.

Caldwell, J. C., P. Caldwell, I. Gajanayake, I. O. Orubuloye, I. Pieris, and P. H. Reddy. 1990. Cultural, Social and Behavioural Determinants of Health and Their Mechanisms: A Report on Related Research Programs. In *What We Know about the Health Transition: The Proceedings of an International Workshop, Canberra, May 1989*. J. C. Caldwell, S. Findley, P. Caldwell, M. G. Santow, W. H. Cosford, J. Braid, and D. Broers-Freeman, eds. Canberra: Australian National University Press.

Cantrelle, P., and T. Locoh. 1990. Cultural and Social Factors Related to Health in West Africa. In *What We Know about the Health Transition: The Proceedings of an International Workshop, Canberra, May 1989*. J. C. Caldwell, S. Findley, P. Caldwell, M. G. Santow, W. H. Cosford, J. Braid, and D. Broers-Freeman, eds. Canberra: Australian National University Press.

Carvajal, M., and P. Burgess. 1978. Socioeconomic Determinants of Fetal and Child Deaths in Latin America: Comparative Study of Bogota, Caracas and Rio de Janeiro. *Social Science and Medicine* 12:3–4C:89–98.

Cebu Study Team. 1991. Underlying and Proximate Determinants of Child Health. *American Journal of Epidemiology* 133:2:185–201.

Cleland, J., and J. van Ginneken. 1988. Maternal Education and Child Survival in Developing Countries: The Search for Pathways of Influence. *Social Science and Medicine* 27:12:1357–68.

Corbett, J. 1989. *Poverty and Sickness: The High Costs of Ill-Health*. IDS Bulletin 20:2. Sussex: Institute of Development Studies.

Cosminsky, S. 1990. Women's Health Care Strategies on a Guatemalan Plantation. In *What We Know about the Health Transition: The Proceedings of an International Workshop, Canberra, May 1989*. J. C. Caldwell, S. Findley, P. Caldwell, M. G. Santow, W. H. Cosford, J. Braid, and D. Broers-Freeman, eds. Canberra: Australian National University Press.

Crook, N., R. Ramasubban, and B. Singh. 1991. A Multi-Dimensional Approach to the Social Analysis of the Health Transition in Bombay. In *The Measurement of Health Transition Concepts*. A. Hill and J. Cleland, eds. Canberra: Australian National University Press.

Das Gupta, M. 1990. Death Clustering, Maternal Education and the Determinants of Child Mortality in Rural Punjab, India. In *What We Know about the Health Transition: The Proceedings of an International Workshop, Canberra,*

May 1989. J. C. Caldwell, S. Findley, P. Caldwell, M. G. Santow, W. H. Cosford, J. Braid, and D. Broers-Freeman, eds. Canberra: Australian National University Press.

DaVanzo, J., and P. Gertler. 1990. *Household Production of Health: A Microeconomic Perspective on Health Transitions.* Rand Note N–3014-RC, CA. Santa Monica, Calif.: Rand Corporation.

Dubos, R. 1961. *Mirage of Health.* New York: Anchor Books.

———. 1965. *Man Adapting.* New Haven: Yale University Press.

Ewbank, D., and S. Preston. 1990. Personal Health Behavior and the Decline of Infant and Child Mortality: The United States, 1900–1930. In *What We Know about the Health Transition: The Proceedings of an International Workshop, Canberra, May 1989.* J. C. Caldwell, S. Findley, P. Caldwell, M. G. Santow, W. H. Cosford, J. Braid, and D. Broers-Freeman, eds. Canberra: Australian National University Press.

Farah. A. A., and S. Preston. 1982. Child Mortality Differentials in Sudan. *Population and Development Review* 8:2:365–83.

Feachem, R. G. 1985. The Role of Water Supply and Sanitation in Reducing Mortality in China, Costa Rica, Kerala State (India) and Sri Lanka. In *Good Health at Low Cost.* S. B. Halstead, J. Walsh, and K. Warren, eds. New York: Rockefeller Foundation.

———. 1990. *Adult Mortality.* Presentation at the International Clinical Epidemiology Network Meeting. Puebla, Mexico, January.

Feachem, R. G., D. J. Bradley, H. Garelick, and D. D. Mata. 1983. *Sanitation and Disease: Health Aspects of Escreta and Waste Water Management.* Chichester: John Wiley and Sons.

Finerman, R. 1990. Who Benefits from Health Care Decisions? Family Medicine in an Andean Indian Community. In *What We Know about the Health Transition: The Proceedings of an International Workshop, Canberra, May 1989.* J. C. Caldwell, S. Findley, P. Caldwell, M. G. Santow, W. H. Cosford, J. Braid, and D. Broers-Freeman, eds. Canberra: Australian National University Press.

Foster, G. M. 1984. Anthropological Research and Perspectives on Health Problems in Developing Countries. *Social Science and Medicine* 18:10:847–54.

Frenk, Julio, Jose L. Bobadilla, Jaime Sepulvida, and Maliaquias Lopez Cervanto. 1989. Health Transition in Middle Income Countries: New Challenges for Health Care. *Health Policy and Planning* 4:1:29–39.

Ghana Health Assessment Project Team. 1981. A Quantitative Method of Assessing the Health Impact of Different Diseases in Less Developed Countries. *International Journal of Epidemiology* 10:1:73–80.

Good, C. 1987. *Ethnomedical Systems in Africa.* New York: Guilford Press.

Grosse, R. N. 1980. Interrelation between Health and Population: Observations Derived from Field Experiences. *Social Science and Medicine* 12(C):99–120.

Haines, M. R., and R. C. Avery. 1982. Differential Infant and Child Mortality in Costa Rica: 1968–1973. *Population Studies* 36:31–43.

Halstead, S. B., J. Walsh, and K. Warren, eds. 1985. *Good Health at Low Cost.* New York: Rockefeller Foundation.

Handwerker, W. P. 1986. *Culture and Reproduction.* Boulder, Colo.: Westview Press.

Hardiman, M. 1986. People's Involvement in Health and Medical Care. In *Community Participation, Social Development and the State*. J. Midgley, ed. London: Methuen.

Heggenhougen, K. 1991. Perceptions of Health Care Options and Therapy Seeking Behavior. In *Measurement of Health Transition Concepts*. A. Hill and J. Cleland, eds. Canberra: Australian National University Press.

Janzen, J. M. 1978. The Comparative Study of Medical Systems as Changing Social Systems. *Social Science and Medicine* 12:2B:121–33.

———. 1990. Ngoma and the Social Reproduction of Health: Affliction and Ritual Therapy in Central and Southern Africa. In *What We Know about the Health Transition: The Proceedings of an International Workshop, Canberra, May 1989*. J. C. Caldwell, S. Findley, P. Caldwell, M. G. Santow, W. H. Cosford, J. Braid, and D. Broers-Freeman, eds. Canberra: Australian National University Press.

Johansson, S. R. 1990. Cultural Influences on Morbidity and Mortality: Paradigm Shifts, New Perspectives and Cultural Programs for the Management of Health and Longevity. In *What We Know about the Health Transition: Proceedings of an International Workshop, Canberra, May 1989*. J. C. Caldwell, S. Findley, P. Caldwell, M. G. Santow, W. H. Cosford, J. Braid, and D. Broers-Freeman, eds. Canberra: Australian National University Press.

Kleinman, A. 1980. *Patients and Healers in the Context of Culture*. Berkeley: University of California Press.

Lipton, M., and E. deKadt. 1988. *Agriculture—Health Linkages*. Geneva: World Health Organization.

Longhurst, R. 1984. *The Energy Trap: Work, Nutrition, and Child Malnutrition in Northern Nigeria*. Cornell University International Nutrition Monograph Series No. 13. Ithaca, N.Y.: Cornell University Press.

Manton, K. G., J. E. Dowd, and M. A. Woodbury. 1986. Conceptual and Measurement Issues in Assessing Disability Cross-Nationally: Analysis of a WHO-Sponsored Survey of the Disablement Process in Indonesia. *Journal of Cross-Cultural Gerontology* 1:339–62.

Martorell, R., and R. Sharma. 1985. Trends in Nutrition, Food Supply and Infant Mortality Rates. In *Good Health at Low Cost*. S. B. Halstead, J. Walsh, and K. Warren, eds. New York: Rockefeller Foundation.

McKeown, T. 1976. *The Modern Rise of Populations*. New York: Academic Press.

Millard, A. V., A. E. Ferguson, and S. Khaila. 1990. Agricultural Development and Malnutrition in Developing Countries: A Causal Model of Child Mortality. In *What We Know about the Health Transition: The Proceedings of an International Workshop, Canberra, May 1989*. J. C. Caldwell, S. Findley, P. Caldwell, M. G. Santow, W. H. Cosford, J. Braid, and D. Broers-Freeman, eds. Canberra: Australian National University Press.

Morley, D., J. E. Rohde, and G. Williams, eds. 1983. *Practicing Health for All*. Oxford: Oxford University Press.

Mosley, W. H., and L. C. Chen. 1984. An Analytic Framework for the Study of Child Survival in Developing Countries. In *Child Survival: Strategies for Research*. W. H. Mosley and L. C. Chen, eds. *Population and Development Review*, Supplement to vol. 10. New York: The Population Council.

Nag, M. 1990. Political Awareness as a Factor in Accessibility of Health Services:

A Case Study of Rural Kerala and West Bengal. In *What We Know about the Health Transition: The Proceedings of an International Workshop, Canberra, May 1989.* J. C. Caldwell, S. Findley, P. Caldwell, M. G. Santow, W. H. Cosford, J. Braid, and D. Broers-Freeman, eds. Canberra: Australian National University Press.

Nathan, R. P. 1988. *Social Science in Government: Uses and Misues.* New York: Basic Books.

Nations, M. K., and M. F. Farias. 1990. Jeitinha Brasileiro: Cultural Creativity and Making the Medical System Work for Poor Brazilians. In *What We Know about the Health Transition: The Proceedings of an International Workshop, Canberra, May 1989.* J. C. Caldwell, S. Findley, P. Caldwell, M. G. Santow, W. H. Cosford, J. Braid, and D. Broers-Freeman, eds. Canberra: Australian National University Press.

Omran, A. 1971. The Epidemiology of Population Change. *Milbank Memorial Fund Quarterly* 49:509–38.

Panikar, P.G.K., and C. R. Soman. 1984. *Health Status of Kerala: The Paradox of Economic Backwardness and Health Development.* Trivandrum: Centre for Development Studies.

Pison, Gilles, Monique Lefebre, Catherine Enel, and Jean-Francois Trape. 1989. *L'influence des Changements Sanitaires sur L'evolution de la Mortalite: Le Case de Mlomp (Senegal) depuis 50 Ans.* Dossiers et Recherches No. 26. Paris: INED (Institut National d'Etudes Demographiques).

Reddy, P. H. 1989. Epidemiological Transition in India. In *Population Transition in India.* S. N. Singh, M. K. Premi, P. S. Bhatia, and Ashish Bose, eds. Indian Association for the Study of Population. Delhi, India: BR Publishing Co.

Rodgers, G. B. 1979. Income and Inequality as Determinants of Mortality: An International Cross-Sectional Analysis. *Population Studies* 33(2), July.

Rosenfield, P. 1990. The Social Determinants of Tropical Diseases. In *Tropical and Geographical Medicine.* 2d ed. K. S. Warren and A. F. Mahmond, eds. New York: McGraw-Hill.

Rosenzweig, M. R., and T. P. Schultz. 1981. *Child Mortality and Fertility in Colombia: Individual and Community Effects.* Center Discussion Paper No. 380. New Haven, Conn.: Economic Growth Center, Yale University.

Rule, J. 1978. *Insight and Social Betterment: A Preface to Applied Social Science.* New York: Oxford University Press.

Ruzicka, L., and P. Kane. 1990. Health Transition: The Course of Morbidity and Mortality. In *What We Know about the Health Transition: The Proceedings of an International Workshop, Canberra, May 1989.* J. C. Caldwell, S. Findley, P. Caldwell, M. G. Santow, W. H. Cosford, J. Braid, and D. Broers-Freeman, eds. Canberra: Australian National University Press.

Schultz, T. 1985. *Household Economic and Community Variables as Determinants of Mortality.* Proceedings of the International Population Conference, Florence. Liege: Ordina Publications.

Simons, J. 1989. Cultural Dimensions of the Mother's Contribution to Child Survival. In *Selected Readings in the Cultural, Social and Behavioral Determinants of Health.* Health Transition Series No. 1. J. C. Caldwell and G. Santow, eds. Canberra: Australian National University Press.

Strauss, J. 1988. *The Effects of Household and Community Characteristics on the Nutrition of Preschool Children: Evidence from Rural Cote d'Ivoire.* LSMS Working Paper No. 40. Washington, D.C.: World Bank.

Streatfield, K., and M. Singarimbun. 1986. *Social Factors Affecting the Use of Childhood Immunization in Yogyakarta.* Population Studies Center Report Series No. 44. Yogyakarta, Indonesia: Gadja Mada University.

Sushama, P. N. 1990. Social Context of Health Behavior in Kerala. In *What We Know about the Health Transition: The Proceedings of an International Workshop, Canberra, May 1989.* J. C. Caldwell, S. Findley, P. Caldwell, M. G. Santow, W. H. Cosford, J. Braid, and D. Broers-Freeman, eds. Canberra: Australian National University Press.

Tekce, B., and F. C. Shorter. 1984. Determinants of Child Mortality: A Study of Squatter Settlements in Jordan. In *Child Survival: Strategies for Research.* W. H. Mosley and L. C. Chen, eds. *Population and Development Review,* Supplement to vol. 10. New York: The Population Council.

Van de Walle, E., and F. Van de Walle. 1990. The Private and the Public Child. In *What We Know about the Health Transition: The Proceedings of an International Workshop, Canberra, May 1989.* J. C. Caldwell, S. Findley, P. Caldwell, M. G. Santow, W. H. Cosford, J. Braid, and D. Broers-Freeman, eds. Canberra: Australian National University Press.

Visaria, L. 1990. Socio-Cultural Determinants of Health in Rural Gujarat: Results of a Longitudinal Study. In *What We Know about the Health Transition: The Proceedings of an International Workshop, Canberra, May 1989.* J. C. Caldwell, S. Findley, P. Caldwell, M. G. Santow, W. H. Cosford, J. Braid, and D. Broers-Freeman, eds. Canberra: Australian National University Press.

Walsh, J. A. 1985. Estimating the Burden of Illness in the Tropics. In *Tropical and Geographical Medicine.* K. S. Warren and A.A.F. Mahmond, eds. Singapore: McGraw-Hill.

Ware, H. 1984. Effects of Maternal Education, Women's Roles and Child Care on Child Mortality. In *Child Survival: Strategies for Research.* W. H. Mosley and L. C. Chen, eds. *Population and Development Review,* Supplement to vol., 10. New York: The Population Council.

Woods, R. 1990. The Role of Public Health Initiatives in the Nineteenth-Century Mortality Decline. In *What We Know about the Health Transition: The Proceedings of an International Workshop, Canberra, May 1989.* J. C. Caldwell, S. Findley, P. Caldwell, M. G. Santow, W. H. Cosford, J. Braid, and D. Broers-Freeman, eds. Canberra: Australian National University Press.

PART I
THE CONCEPTUALIZATION OF BEHAVIORAL CHANGE

1

An Anthropological Approach to Social Science Research on the Health Transition

NORMA C. WARE, NICHOLAS A. CHRISTAKIS, AND
ARTHUR KLEINMAN

When we use the term "health transition," we refer to the dramatic decrease in mortality that the world has seen over the course of the twentieth century, and to the social forces that figure as both causes and consequence of this transition. Also part of the health transition is a change in the distribution of causes of death and in the prevalence of different types of illness. Acute infectious diseases now represent less of the burden of morbidity in developing countries than before, while the proportion of chronic illness (e.g., heart disease, cancer) is on the rise. At the same time, urbanization and other aspects of modernizing social change are bringing with them an increase in psychological disorders and behavioral disorders, such as substance abuse, child abuse, depression and anxiety disorders, and suicide. Thus, we see that the health transition has three essential aspects: (1) an increase in life expectancy, (2) epidemiological changes in the patterning of illness worldwide, and (3) a growth in psychological and behavioral pathology.

Up to now, much of the research designed to illuminate social influences on the health transition has focused upon the impact of macro-level social processes—improved education, urbanization, mass communication, economic development. Here we argue for the importance of incorporating microsocial variables—variables representing patterns of behavior in local cultural settings—into social science research on the health transition. The argument is based on the proposition that events at the local level serve to mediate the effects of large-scale socioeconomic change upon health outcomes. It follows from this premise that any adequate representation of the nature and determinants of the health transition must account for the effects of microsocial processes.[1]

As a means of presenting this argument, we have chosen to examine the notion of illness behavior, a descriptive and analytical category essential to the study of changes in health status. The aims of the discussion are threefold: (1) to use illness behavior as a conceptual framework for organizing data on cultural variation in the ways people think about and respond to illness; (2) to demonstrate the importance of including microsocial variables in social research on the health transition by documenting cross-cultural differences in illness behavior; and (3) to outline a few of the implications for research and policy formulation that a focus on illness behavior suggests.

ILLNESS BEHAVIOR

Illness behavior is defined here as that constellation of activities and beliefs exhibited by an individual and his or her social circle in response to bodily indications perceived as symptoms (Mechanic 1978).

In a given individual or social network, illness behavior involves the definition of symptoms, the monitoring of the body (to see if the symptoms change or progress), and remedial or "treatment" action, that is, utilization of lay or professional help to rectify the perceived abnormality. The series of activities aimed at securing treatment for the illness is, for present purposes, termed "help-seeking." Help may be sought from a number of different sources in an individual's social network, including friends, family, folk healers, and biomedical professionals. Home care, or treatment administered by sick persons themselves, their families, and their friends, is also part of the help-seeking process.

Help-seeking culminates in the formulation of a treatment plan, or regimen. The extent to which the treatment plan is carried out by the patient and his or her family is referred to as the degree of compliance.

Illness behavior is also influenced by explanatory models of illness. The term "explanatory model" refers to the patient's and family's conceptions of the nature of a particular illness episode, its causes and effects, expected and/or desired treatment, and apprehensions about the outcome. Explanatory models are grounded in culturally defined systems of meaning, crystallizing out of local beliefs about the nature of the body, of suffering, and of the person. Cultural categories that organize various types of illness and methods of treatment also inform explanatory models.

Explanatory models find expression in particular episodes of illness. They rationalize decisions about what is most at stake and what sort of treatment action should be undertaken. Thus, among North Americans, patients may interpret hypertension as a result of "too much tension" rather than high blood pressure. Consequently, patients who feel tense believe they have the condition, while those who do not frequently decline to comply with medical treatment regimens out of a belief that they are not affected (Blumhagen 1980).

All aspects of illness behavior vary with culture. Symptoms are perceived, interpreted, and acted upon differently by people in different cultural contexts, resulting in highly distinctive experiences of illness. The following review of research literature on illness behavior in developing societies documents local-level variation in symptom definition, help-seeking, compliance, and explanatory models.

CULTURE AND SYMPTOM DEFINITION

Recognition of symptoms of indicators of illness is essential to the initiation of help-seeking and treatment. Whether or not particular bodily changes will be identified as symptoms, however, is a function of local cultural definitions of disease. To illustrate, let us consider the case of diarrheal illness.

One researcher reports that among rural Sinhalese in Sri Lanka, diarrhea may be defined both as a form of illness and as a sign of imbalance or transition, depending upon the circumstances. The occurrence of diarrhea during natural transitions in the life of an infant (teething, walking, weaning) is interpreted as a normal response to developmental change—a "trouble," not an illness. Consequently, medical intervention is usually viewed as unnecessary in cases occurring under the age of three unless more serious complaints (such as fever, vomiting) are also involved (Nichter 1988). The tendency to define diarrhea as a natural consequence of growing up rather than as an illness requiring treatment has also been observed in other parts of South Asia (Mull and Mull 1988), in Central and South America (Escobar, Salazar, and Chuy 1983; Kendall, Foote, and Martorell 1983), and in Africa (DeZoysa, Carson, Feachem, Kirkwood, Lindsay-Smith, and Loewenson 1984; Maina-Ahlberg 1979). Likewise, in an earlier study in South India, observers noted that children with diarrhea who became severely dehydrated were often not brought for medical treatment. Subsequent interviews with families in the region revealed that although diarrhea itself was considered an individual abnormality that could be appropriately treated using biomedicine, diarrhea accompanied by what (in biomedical terms) are symptoms of severe dehydration (e.g., sunken eyes, sunken fontanelle) was seen not as an illness but as a form of pollution requiring ritual purification. A therapeutic intervention consistent with biomedical and local cultural interpretations was then devised (Lozoff, Kamath, and Feldman 1975).

An awareness of cultural variability in symptom definition also helps to illuminate the pattern of "illness neglect" that has been identified in various developing world settings.

A number of authors have argued that in areas where mortality rates are high and people are generally poor, a fatalistic attitude toward illness prevails. Life is not as highly valued as it is elsewhere, the argument suggests, and people tend to resign themselves to illness, interpreting it as divine punishment or unavoidable suffering that must simply be endured (Cassidy 1980; Scheper-Hughes 1984; Scrimshaw 1978).

An awareness of cultural variation in symptom definition suggests, however, that so-called neglect of the sick may stem not from fatalism, but from (among other things) the definition of particular bodily changes as acceptable, or even normal, in a given setting. In fact, the notion of fatalistic resignation to disease in the Third World has been rejected by other investigators as a form of blaming the victim. Nations and Rebhun, for example, have convincingly countered claims of maternal neglect in Northeastern Brazil by showing that mothers go to considerable lengths to obtain care for their sick children and grieve profoundly when a child dies (Nations and Rebhun 1988).[2]

HELP-SEEKING

The array of resources from which a sick individual seeks help may be grouped into three overlapping categories, or sectors: (1) the *popular sector*, consisting of families, members of social networks, and patients themselves; (2) the *folk sector*, consisting of traditional healers, and (3) the *professional sector*, meaning practitioners of biomedicine (Good 1987; Kleinman 1980). Our discussion of cultural variation in help-seeking is organized in terms of these three sectors.

The Popular Sector

Where access to professional healers is limited, as it is in much of the developing world, sick people tend to rely heavily on themselves, their families, and other members of their social circle for care.

In examining the dynamics of help-seeking in the popular sector, a number of researchers have chosen to focus on home treatment. In fact, the available data suggest that there may be considerable cultural variation in the extent to which home treatment is used initially or exclusively in coping with illness. Studies carried out in East Asia, Central America, and West Africa showed that 90 percent of urban Taiwanese (Kleinman 1980), 57 percent of poor Salvadorans (Ferguson 1986), and more than 70 percent of mothers in Burkina Faso (Sauerborn, Nougata, and Diesfeld 1989) turned first to home health care. However, other investigators have found the proportion of illness episodes treatment at home to be considerably lower—39 percent in a study in Guatemala (Cosminsky

1987), 29 percent in Sri Lanka (Caldwell, 1989), and 20 percent in Ethiopia (Kloos, Etea, Degefa, Aga, Solomon, Abera, Abegaz, and Belemo 1987).

It is important to recognize that home treatment is usually not the only form of care sought in response to a given illness episode. In most cases, home care is followed by consultation with traditional healers and/or biomedical practitioners. This pattern is illustrated by the results of a recent study of health service utilization in Kathmandu, Nepal, in which patients were found to turn first to home remedies, then to traditional healers, and only finally to biomedical health services for treatment (Subedi 1989).

A paper synthesizing the results of four different studies carried out in isolated rural areas of India and Nepal provides useful comparative data on patterns of self-care in two different developing countries. The proportion of ill individuals reporting use of self-care either alone or in combination with professional treatment over a two-week period ranged from 19 to 42 percent (Parker, Shah, Alexander, and Neumann 1979).[3] Reliance on self-care was generally lower in Nepal than in the Indian research sites, but it did not vary by age or sex in any of the studies reported. It is interesting to note that data from North and South India revealed a significant decline in self-care practices over the course of a 10-week period. Reported use of self-care tended to be slightly higher in areas at a greater distance from professional services. Variation in recourse to self-care by type and severity of complaint was also demonstrated.

Finally, it must be recognized that self-medication with pharmaceuticals is becoming an increasingly important aspect of home care. Regardless of how we choose to explain this phenomenon,[4] western drugs are growing in popularity in many developing countries. Easily available from pharmacists or even local lay personnel (Whyte 1991), these medicines are often misused for self-treatment by the general population, who consume then without benefit of knowledgeable direction or advice (Ferguson 1986; Haak and Hardon 1988). The widespread distribution of pharmaceuticals is promoted by western (and indigenous) drug companies, whose primary interest lies, generally speaking, in maximizing profit.

Social networks are another component of the popular sector from which help is sought in times of illness. In the process of responding to an illness episode, the social network of the affected individual may influence diagnosis of the condition, choice of healers, and provision of care. An entire community may become involved, for example, in speculation about the nature and cause of a given condition, especially when the patient is a child (Crandon 1983). One author coined the term "therapy management group" in an attempt to convey the central importance of the social network for decisionmaking and therapeutic activity in

Lower Zaire (Janzen 1978). Therapy management groups are also important in South India, where their purpose is not only to facilitate optimal treatment but also to manage the distribution of resources. Considerable overt and covert conflict is often involved in this process.[5]

A study of traditional healers in Singapore found that 57 percent of patients using these services were referred to them by family or friends. In the investigation of health services utilization in Nepal cited previously, consultation with family or friends was found to be associated with a longer period between the onset of illness and the decision to seek medical help (Subedi 1989). Finally, for an illustration of the extensive role social networks can play in the provision of care, we may look to data from rural Brazil, where informal adoption of desperate or dying children by members of the community has been reported to be relatively commonplace (Scheper-Hughes 1987).

Another important function of the social network is the provision of social support, which has repeatedly been shown to be related to health status. We know, for example, that the risk of health problems is higher for individuals whose social relationships are few and their quality poor (House, Landis, and Umberson 1988). When social support is lacking, emotional distress may be manifested as bodily complaints. This process has been described in a study of Havik Brahmin women in South Kanara, India, where it is argued that in the absence of adequate social support, personal, social, and organic distress are expressed in a somatic idiom (Nichter 1981).

It is important to emphasize that care received from resources in the popular sector of not necessarily inferior to professional treatment. A mother who administers oral rehydration therapy to a child with diarrhea and dehydration is providing care that is eminently appropriate and often life saving. Other forms of popular treatment may involve dietary changes and special foods, traditional herbs and medicines, cupping and massage, religious practices, and biomedical interventions.

Folk and Professional Sectors

The steady advance of western biomedicine in developing societies means that traditional and cosmopolitan healing systems now coexist in many regions of the world. Thus, the study of help-seeking from folk and professional sources becomes in large part the study of choices between traditional and biomedical practitioners.[6] A number of different types of factors help to shape such choices. Three of these will be considered here: the type of illness involved, the perceived cause of the illness, and the accessibility of services.

Often, in situations of medical pluralism, a classification system develops to specify which types of complaints should be treated by a traditional healer and which through the use of biomedicine. A study of the use of traditional Chinese medicine in Singapore, for example, showed that this form of treatment was strongly preferred for rheumatism, fractures, menstrual irregularities, and anemia. Chinese medicine was also significantly preferred for diarrhea, worm infestations, influenza, and constipation (Ho Lun, and Ny 1984). In Nigeria, in contrast, traditional healers have been found to be preferred for psychiatric illness, fractures, snake bites, and convulsions (Nnadi and Kabat 1984).

Choices among healers in the folk or professional sectors may also be guided by notions of illness etiology. For example, in rural Ghana, local categories of disease causation define specific illnesses as the result of actions of supernatural agents, natural agents, or both. A study of help-seeking patterns carried out in this region showed that biomedical practitioners were consulted more often than traditional healers for illnesses considered to have natural causes, while for conditions attributed to supernatural forces, the reverse was true (Fosu 1981).

To cite a second and rather different case, researchers studying traditional beliefs and practices related to diarrhea in rural Pakistan found certain types of diarrhea to be represented as particular "folk" illnesses with ascribed causes such as fallen fontanelle or exposure to "envious glances" (Mull and Mull 1988). A systematic comparison of the types of care sought for these two forms of diarrheal illness revealed a clear relationship between attribution to "folk causes" and a preference for traditional healers.

The relative accessibility of traditional biomedical practitioners also plays an important role in determining what type of healer will be consulted. Accessibility is determined by a number of factors, including distance, transportation, waiting time, linguistic barriers, and cost.

In a study of healer choice in a Mexican village, for example, 58 percent of subjects cited problems of access, such as lack of money or transportation, as their reason for deciding not to consult a physician (Young 1981a, 1981b). Similarly, research on physician use in Northern Nigeria revealed that per capita utilization of local government health dispensaries declined steadily as distance to the facility increased.[7] A recent study of malaria treatment in Africa pointed to lack of access to medications as a major factor in explaining why mothers did not use anti-malarial drugs for episodes of fever in their children and themselves (Glik et al. 1989).

The fact that choices are made between traditional or professional practitioners does not mean, however, that the folk and professional sectors are mutually exclusive. People may seek treatment from both types of health care systems concurrently or sequentially in the course of a single illness episode, acting out of the belief that traditional healing and biomedicine represent complementary, rather than competing, approaches to health care.

COMPLIANCE WITH TREATMENT

The research literature reporting influences on compliance with treatment in Third World settings identifies different factors in different cultural contexts.[8] For example, failure to achieve the anticipated response emerged as a major consideration in an investigation of oral rehydration solution (ORS) treatment of diarrhea in North India. Forty percent of study subjects who had tried ORS for diarrheal illness reported that they would not use it again because it did not bring about the effect they expected, namely, cessation of the diarrhea (Bentley 1988). Of course, ORS merely replaces lost fluid; it does not treat the diarrhea itself.

A recent study designed to uncover the reasons behind widespread noncompliance with medical regimens among leprosy patients in Pakistan illustrates the impact of cultural and social factors upon adherence to treatment (Mull, Wood, Gans, and Mull 1989). In this research, a model of compliance that took health beliefs, duration and complexity of treatment, relief of symptoms, and quality of the doctor-patient relationship into account nonetheless proved to be inadequate in that it failed to incorporate a recognition of the social stigma attached to this disease. Leprosy patients who participated in the research reported having been shunned by their neighbors (34 percent), rejected by their families (27 percent), fired from their jobs (19 percent), forced to leave their homes (14 percent), and/or unable to find marriage partners (11 percent). The fact that the majority (54 percent) of noncompliant subjects who were questioned denied having the disease (precluding, of course, the necessity for treatment) is interpreted by the investigators as an understandable response to these kinds of experiences.

In their analysis of fatalism, neglect, and childhood illness in Northeastern Brazil, Nations and Rebhun (1988) describe the local ethical systems that help to guide families in making the decision to discontinue treatment for a child who is considered terminally ill. Severity of symptoms, available resources for treatment, the anticipated burden on family resources that administration of the treatment represents, and the quality of life the child is likely to enjoy if he or she survives are some of the criteria used by parents, in consultation with traditional healers, in making a "decision for death." The authors make a point of articulating the similarities between the Brazilian folk system and its analogue in professional biomedicine.

The data from Pakistan and Brazil make it clear that to construe compliance only as a moral imperative emanating from the biomedical establishment is to miss the important influences of popular moralities upon this aspect of illness behavior. Patients, families, and communities routinely invoke local meanings to evaluate the effectiveness of treatment. Much more needs to be known about how cultural beliefs influence decisions such as whether or not to return to a particular caregiver, where else to go for treatment, or when a particular episode of illness is considered to be over. In short, scientific models of compliance must incorporate a recognition of local moral systems and their behavioral implications, if their purpose is to be well served.

EXPLANATORY MODELS

For an especially clear illustration of cultural variability in explanatory models of illness, we may look again to the data on diarrhea. We have seen that under certain circumstances, in particular cultural contexts, symptoms of diarrhea may not be defined as an indication of illness. In most instances, however, diarrhea is interpreted as illness, and its occurrence is attributed to a wide variety of possible causes. These are summarized in a useful review article by Weiss (1988) to include the following: (1) imbalance of heat and cold in the body (reported in Northeastern Brazil, Honduras, North and South India), (2) bad breast milk (reported in the Philippines, Zimbabwe, Bangladesh), (3) worms (especially prevalent in Latino cultures), (4) supernatural causes (reported in Brazil, South India), and (5) immoral conduct, such as sexual infidelity on the part of an afflicted child's parents (reported in Africa).

A number of different explanatory models for a given illness may also coexist within a single cultural region. Thus, in the study of noncompliance in leprosy patients cited previously, the disease was variously attributed to (1) conflicts or imbalances between hot and cold foods in the diet (47 percent of study subjects), (2) physical causes (such as "bad blood" or "germs"—28 percent), (3) environmental forces (cold weather, hot weather, winds—20 percent), (4) emotional and magical causes (evil eye, being cursed, feeling proud or angry—3 percent), and (5) the will of God (16 percent) (Mull, Wood, Gans, and Mull 1989).

The culturally specific nature of explanatory models becomes especially apparent when a translation between cultures is attempted. Consider the case of a Samoan family, recent immigrants to Hawaii, who had difficulty making sense of western physicians' diagnosis of diabetes mellitus in their daughter (Krantzler 1987). It was explained that the patient had a problem with "sugar." The parents concluded from this that inadequate sugar was the cause of the difficulty, and they responded by ignoring the recommendation for insulin injections and supplementing their daughter's diet with sweets. Western physicians interpreted this as deliberate disregard for medical care.

The data on the impact of notions of illness etiology upon help-seeking suggest a certain consistency between the type of cause to which an illness is ascribed and the type of healer consulted. Other research in developing societies, in contrast, points to an apparent inconsistency. For example, a study of the health behavior of traditionally oriented and more modern-oriented women in a Mexican community (McClain 1977) showed that while study subjects with both orientations tended to conceptualize disease etiology and process in terms of traditional cognitive models, traditionally oriented women participated partially, and modern-oriented women fully, in the biomedical system. The author concludes from these findings that behavioral change proceeds faster than cognitive change, with respect to biomedical care. She attributes this to the fact that biomedical practitioners typically do not discuss disease etiology and process with their clients, concluding that "Modern medical practices and materials are available as alternatives to traditional counterparts, but medical cognitive models remain effectively hidden from observation, and therefore, from acceptance" (p. 341). This interpretation has been corroborated by the results of more recent research (Cosminsky and Scrimshaw 1980).

IMPLICATIONS FOR RESEARCH AND POLICY

A number of significant gaps in our knowledge of illness behavior in the developing world remain to be filled by additional research. Among these are (1) help-seeking patterns that combine resources from the popular, folk, and professional sectors, (2) factors affecting compliance with treatment, (3) illness behavior in chronic illness, and (4) the ways in which particular types of illness behavior work to influence health status.

A few of the factors that have been shown to influence help-seeking in the popular, folk, and professional sectors have been outlined here. Much remains to be understood, however, of the relative significance of these and other factors in particular cultural settings, and of the dynamics of the processes involved. What does the help-seeking process look like "on the ground"? How do particular individuals or families weigh the various considerations involved at each step, and how does this differ across cultural settings? What regularities can be identified in the ways people combine resources from different health care sectors? These kinds of questions are best answered through ethnographic research.

Referral patterns in help-seeking is another area where additional research is needed. Who makes referrals to whom? Are certain individuals or types of individuals especially influential in particular societies with respect to healer choice? What part do social networks play in the referral process?

Compliance with treatment is an extremely important area for further research. Why do people choose to ignore recommendations for treatment? How can instructions be presented in a way that maximizes the likelihood of their being followed? What is the role of local systems of ethics in facilitating or complicating compliance? There are only a few of the questions that merit additional attention from social science researchers.

As we have seen, the changing composition of morbidity in the direction of increases in chronic illness is one of the defining characteristics of the health transition. Yet very little is known of the nature of illness behavior in chronic disease in the Third World or of the social factors that affect it. Additional research in this area would do much to illuminate the burden of disability in developing societies. The role of traditional healers in caring for chronically ill individuals is of particular significance here.

Finally, we need to know more about the mechanisms and processes through which illness behavior works to influence health status. What are the relationships between help-seeking patterns and health outcomes for particular illnesses? How are these relationships influenced by other aspects of illness behavior, such as patients' explanatory models? Does compliance with recommended biomedical treatment actually affect outcome? Under what conditions and in what ways?

Turning to health policy, steps should be taken to close the gap between behavioral and cognitive change with respect to the use of biomedical services. As we have seen, research on help-seeking from traditional and biomedical healers suggests that people may avail themselves of medical services without fully understanding them. While this might appear to be a positive development, its undesirable effects—for example, in the form of noncompliance with treatment or inappropriate use of drugs—should also be recognized. People must have a cognitive framework in which to place their experiences with biomedicine if they are to make safe and effective use of professional care. To this end, physicians and other biomedical practitioners working in developing countries should be trained to function not only as clinicians but also as educators who can explain the reasons behind the procedures they use and the treatments they prescribe.

CONCLUSION

Our intention here has been to argue for the necessity of incorporating local-level, cultural variables into social science research on the health transition. By reviewing empirical evidence of cross-cultural differences in illness behavior, we hope to demonstrate that attempts to explain the health transition in terms of its social determinants will prove inadequate unless cultural variation is taken into account. The power and sophistication of social science models of the health transition are likely to be greatly increased when variables representing microsocial processes are included.

We have chosen to present data on illness behavior as a means of making this case. But an illness behavior perspective has other advantages as well. First, the study of illness behavior by definition shifts the direction of our analytical gaze from mortality to morbidity. The fact that this same shift is one of the essential features of the health transition makes illness behavior an excellent conceptual tool for examining changes in health status.

Perhaps more important, however, is the fact that a focus on illness behavior brings a recognition of the importance of suffering, as one aspect of the experience of illness, to the attention of the social science researcher. Suffering merits serious investigation because it is part of what is at stake in human experience worldwide. To neglect suffering in developing countries in the interest of highlighting the burden of mortality is to adopt an inhumane approach to Third World problems— an approach that would be regarded as scandalous if applied in a western context (Farmer and Kleinman 1989). The recognition of human rights in the health care domain requires the legitimization of suffering—the endurance of pain, the daily struggle of coping with chronic disease— as a crucial moral category. The study of illness behavior enables us to acknowledge these other, deeply human, aspects of illness experience (Kleinman 1988).

However, the problem of suffering is a problem of meaning as well as experience—a teleological quest to find moral and existential explanations for one's illness, to answer the question, "Why me?" Anthropological research on health and illness reveals that, of the many and varied systems of healing to be found around the world, only biomedicine systematically excludes the teleological dimensions of suffering from its stipulated domain. And this is, perhaps, the way it should be. For to attempt to apply the tools of the biomedical trade to fundamental questions of meaning and existence is to risk dehumanizing these questions by reducing them to problems of science and technology. Moral and spiritual epistemologies cannot be replaced by scientific models, regardless of their undeniable value in addressing the biological aspects of disease.

Neither should we rely too heavily on social science in this regard. While ethical and psychosocial interpretations are essential components of any comprehensive program of research on health and disease, they too fall short, and necessarily so, in responding to the teleological issues that arise out of the experience of suffering in illness.

This tension between science and teleology is, and will continue to be, central to the dynamics of the health transition as biomedicine continues its advance into the developing world. An anthropological perspective on the processes of social change involved in the transition focuses attention on the significance of local systems of moral and religious knowledge as sources of existential meaning that biomedicine, with all of its healing power, cannot provide.

NOTES

1. For a detailed discussion of this, see N. Christakis, N. Ware, and A. Kleinman, "Illness Behavior and the Health Transition in the Developing World," in *Health and Social Changes in International Perspective*, eds. L. C. Chen, A. M. Kleinman, J. Potter, and N. C. Ware. In Preparation.

2. This is not to suggest that fatalism does not figure in interpretations of illness in the Third World. Rather, where this is the case, fatalistic attributions should be understood in terms of the larger system of meanings in which they are embedded. Similarly, we do not wish to suggest that families cannot be more effective in protecting the health of children. We do claim, however, that entire communities can rarely be justifiably charged with fatalism or negligence when other factors are taken into account.

3. These results are, of course, not strictly comparable, since they were obtained through different studies carried out at different times. Nonetheless, the findings are of interest in that (1) they are based on attempts to assess roughly the same phenomenon, and (2) they offer data from a number of different research sites.

4. Van der Geest and Whyte (1989), for example, choose to explain it in terms of the tangibility and concreteness of pharmaceuticals, which lift the experience of illness out of the ambiguous tangle of social relationships while connoting the power and authority of biomedicine.

5. John Caldwell, personal communication.

6. We recognize that important distinctions among the many different types of healers found around the world are underemphasized in this report. These distinctions have been subsumed under a single heading in order to focus attention on the matter of primary interest for this discussion.

7. Beliefs about the relative effectiveness of traditional and biomedical treatment also play an important role in determining healer choice. For a discussion of the impact of perceived efficacy upon help-seeking in situations of medical pluralism, see Christakis, Ware and Kleinman, "Illness Behavior and the Health Transition in the Developing World," in *Health and Social Change in International Perspective*, eds. L. C. Chen, A. Kleinman, J. Potter, and N. C. Ware. Forthcoming from Oxford University Press, New York.

8. Again, a rigorous demonstration of cross-cultural variation in factors affecting compliance with treatment would require controlling for variables such as type of illness. In the absence of systematically comparable data from different

cultural settings, we may conservatively interpret the relevant findings as suggestive, if not definitive, evidence of cultural differences.

REFERENCES

Bentley, M. D. 1988. The Household Management of Child Diarrhea in Rural Northern India. *Social Science and Medicine* 27:1:75–85.

Blumhagen, D. 1980. Hypertension: A Folk-Illness with a Medical Name. *Culture, Medicine and Psychiatry* 4:197–228.

Caldwell, J. C., I. Gajanayake, P. Caldwell, and I. Peiris. 1989. Sensitization to Illness and the Risk of Death: An Explanation for Sri Lanka's Approach to Good Health for All. *Social Science and Medicine* 28:4:365–79.

Cassidy, C. M. 1980. Benign Neglect and Toddler Malnutrition. In *Social and Biological Predictors of Nutritional Status, Physical Growth, and Neurological Development.* L. S. Greene and R. E. Johnston, eds. New York: Academic Press.

Cosminsky, S. 1987. Women and Health Care on a Guatemalan Plantation. *Social Science and Medicine* 25:10:1163–73.

Cosminsky, S., and M. Scrimshaw. 1980. Medical Pluralism on a Guatemalan Plantation. *Social Science and Medicine* 14B:267–78.

Crandon, L. 1983. Why Susto? *Ethnology* 22:2:153–67.

DeZoysa, I., D. Carson, R. Feachem, B. Kirkwood, E. Lindsay-Smith and R. Loewenson. 1984. Perceptions of Childhood Diarrhea and Its Treatment in Rural Zimbabwe. *Social Science and Medicine* 19:727–34.

Escobar, G. J., E. Salazar, and M. Chuy. 1983. Beliefs Regarding the Etiology and Treatment of Infantile Diarrhea in Lima, Peru. *Social Science and Medicine* 17:1257–69.

Farmer, P., and A. Kleinman. 1989. AIDS and Human Suffering. *Daedalus* (Spring): 135–60.

Ferguson, A. 1986. Commercial Pharmaceutical Medicine and Medicalization: A Case Study from El Salvador. In *The Context of Medicines in Developing Countries, Studies in Pharmaceutical Anthropology.* S. van der Geest and S. R. Whyte, eds. Boston: Kluwer.

Fosu, G. B. 1981. Disease Classification in Rural Ghana: Framework and Implications for Health Behavior. *Social Science and Medicine* 15B:471–82.

Glik, D. C., et al. 1989. Malaria Treatment Practices among Mothers in Guinea. *Journal of Health and Social Behavior* 30:421–35.

Good, C. 1987. *Ethnomedical Systems in Africa.* New York: Guilford Press.

Haak, H., and A. P. Hardon. 1988. Indigenised Pharmaceuticals in Developing Countries: Widely Used, Widely Neglected. *Lancet* 8611 (September 10): 620–21.

Ho, S. C., K. C. Lun, and W. K. Ng. 1984. The Role of Chinese Traditional Medical Practice as a Form of Health Care in Singapore—III. Conditions, Illness Behavior, and Medical Preferences of Patients of Institutional Clinics. *Social Science and Medicine* 18:9:745–52.

House, J. S., K. R. Landis, and D. Umberson. 1988. Social Relationships and Health. *Science* 241:540–45.

Janzen, J. 1978. *The Quest for Therapy in Lower Zaire*. Berkeley: University of California Press.

Kendall, C., D. Foote, and R. Martorell. 1983. Anthropology, Communications and Health: The Mass Media and Health Practices Programs in Honduras. *Human Organization* 42:353–60.

Kleinman, A. 1980. *Patients and Healers in the Context of Culture*. Berkeley: University of California Press.

———. 1988. *The Illness Narratives: Suffering, Healing and the Human Condition*. New York: Basic Books.

Kloos, H., E. Etea, A. Degefa, H. Aga, B. Solomon, K. Abera, A. Abegaz, and G. Belemo. 1987. Illness and Health Behavior in Addis Ababa and Rural Central Ethiopia. *Social Science and Medicine* 25:9:1003–1019.

Krantzler, N. J. 1987. Traditional Medicine as "Medical Neglect": Dilemmas in the case Management of a Samoan Teenager with Diabetes. In *Child Survival*. N. Scheper-Hughes, ed. Boston: D. Reidel.

Lozoff, L. B., D. R. Kamath, and R. A. Feldman. 1975. Infection and Disease in South Indian Families: Beliefs about Childhood Diarrhea. *Human Organization* 34:353–58.

Maina-Ahlberg, B. 1979. Beliefs and Practices concerning the Treatment of Measles and Acute Diarrhea among the Akamba. *Tropical Geographical Medicine* 31:139–48.

McClain, C. 1977. Adaptation in Health Behavior: Modern and Traditional Medicine in a West Mexican Community. *Social Science and Medicine* 11:341–47.

Mechanic, D. 1978. Illness. In *Medical Sociology*. D. Mechanic, ed. New York: Free Press.

Mull, J. D., and D. S. Mull. 1988. Mothers' Concepts of Childhood Diarrhea in Rural Pakistan: What ORT Program Planners Should Know. *Social Science and Medicine* 27:1:53–67.

Mull, J. D., C. S. Wood, L. P. Gans, and D. S. Mull. 1989. Culture and "Compliance" among Leprosy Patients in Pakistan. *Social Science and Medicine* 29:7:799–811.

Nations, M. K., and L. A. Rebhun. 1988. Angels with Wet Wings Won't Fly: Maternal Sentiment in Brazil and the Image of Neglect. *Culture, Medicine and Psychiatry* 12:2:141–200.

Nichter, M. 1981. Idioms of Distress—Alternatives in the Expression of Psychosocial Distress: A Case Study from South India. *Culture, Medicine and Psychiatry* 5:379–408.

———. 1988. From *Aralu* to ORS: Sinhalese Perceptions of Digestion, Diarrhea, and Dehydration. *Social Science and Medicine* 27:1:39–52.

Nnadi, E. E., and H. F. Kabat. 1984. Choosing Health Care Services in Nigeria: A Developing Nation. *Journal of Tropical Medicine and Hygiene* 87:47–51.

Parker, R. L., S. M. Shah, C. A. Alexander, and A. K. Neumann. 1979. Self Care in Rural Areas of India and Nepal. *Culture, Medicine and Psychiatry* 3:3–28.

Sauerborn, R., A. Nougata, and H. J. Diesfeld. 1989. Low Utilization of Community Health Workers: Results from a Household Interview Survey in Burkina Faso. *Social Science and Medicine* 29:10:1163–74.

Scheper-Hughes, N. 1984. Infant Mortality and Infant Care: Cultural and Economic Constraints on Nurturing in Northeast Brazil. *Social Science and Medicine* 19:5:535–46.

———. 1987. Culture, Scarcity and Maternal Thinking: Mother Love and Child Death in Northeastern Brazil. In *Child Survival*. N. Scheper-Hughes, ed. Boston: D. Reidel.

Scrimshaw, N. 1978. Infant Mortality and Behavior in the Regulation of Family Size. *Population and Development Review* 4:383–403.

Subedi, J. 1989. Modern Health Services and Health Care Behavior: A Survey in Kathmandu, Nepal. *Journal of Health and Social Behavior* 30:412–30.

van der Geest, S., and S. R. Whyte. 1989. The Charm of Medicines: Metaphors and Metonyms. *Medical Anthropology Quarterly* 3:4:345–67.

Weiss, M. 1988. Cultural Models of Diarrheal Illness: Conceptual Framework and Review. *Social Science and Medicine* 27:1:5–16.

Whyte, S. R. 1992. Privatization of Health Care in Eastern Uganda. In *Structural Adjustment and the State of Uganda*. H. B. Hansen and M. Twaddle, eds. London: James Croom, forthcoming.

Young, J. C. 1981a. *Medical Choice in a Mexican Village*. New Brunswick, N.J.: Rutgers University Press.

———. 1981b. Non-Use of Physicians: Methodological Approaches, Policy Implications, and the Utility of Decision Models. *Social Science and Medicine* 15B:499–506.

2

Behavioral Medicine, Health Behavior, and Health Maintenance Strategies: Applicability to Disease Prevention in the Developing World

STEPHEN M. WEISS

The term "behavioral medicine" reflects the intent of those concerned with mind-body issues "to develop and integrate the biomedical and behavioral sciences' knowledge and techniques relevant to health and illness and to apply this knowledge and these techniques to prevention diagnosis treatment and rehabilitation" (Schwartz and Weiss 1978). The scientists and clinicians responsible for creating this interdisciplinary approach recognized that the collective expertise of many disciplines would be necessary to comprehend the multifaceted nature of the health problems currently facing the nation.

Since the early 1970s, when *lifestyle* was first cited as a major ingredient in national health care planning (Lalonde 1974), strategies to alter human behavior as a means of changing health status have received increasing attention by those concerned with national health policy in industrialized countries. The preventive and behavioral medicine scientific communities have also directed considerable attention and energy to this issue. For example, funding of "health and behavior" research at the U.S. National Institutes of Health has quintupled over the past 13 years, from $42 million in 1976 (Weiss 1982) to over $300 million in 1990.

The Framingham Heart Study (e.g., Kannel, Dawber, Kagan, Revotski, and Stokes 1961) and the Alameda County Study (Belloc and Breslow 1972), among others, have established strong epidemiologic foundations for the association between behavior and health, identifying smoking, diet, exercise, obesity, and blood pressure regulation as key determinants of cardiovascular health and longevity. Our ability to successfully cope with the stressors in our daily world has also received considerable attention in recent years as a potential major determinant of health status.

During the past 10 years, disease prevention/health promotion programs in schools, communities, and worksites have proliferated in exponential fashion in the United States. Similar programs are also rapidly taking hold in other countries in the industrialized world. For example, nearly 2,000 corporations in the United States offer some form of health promotion for their employees. Health planners and economists are also beginning to recognize the potential of lifestyle modification as a means of preventing illness and, therefore, bringing down the escalating costs of a health care system based on curing disease.

Although the behavioral changes required to effect positive health outcomes appear outwardly simple and straightforward, the frustrations of the hundreds of scientists attempting to change these behaviors attest to the underlying complexity of the task. These frustrations have forced researchers to cast a broader net in seeking explanations for their failures both to successfully change behaviors and to maintain those changes once they have been initiated. This search has typically led to areas beyond the usual boundaries of any given researcher's discipline; the many disciplines concerned with health and behavior have begun to join forces in an effort to address these problems at each of the various levels at which they present themselves.

A relatively straightforward, measurable, quantifiable behavior such as smoking, for example, has shown itself to be particularly refractory to the intensive information bombardment regarding risks of cancer, heart disease, and respiratory disease. Although such information may be necessary, it is clearly not sufficient to have a meaningful impact on the prevalence of smoking. Scientists who originally conceived of smoking as a psychological/behavioral problem have begun to appreciate the contributions of genetics, early development, and social and cultural determinants. Recognizing the multifactorial nature of the problem has led to consideration of multidimensional approaches to its resolution. This has paved the way for multifaceted therapies that employ the combined expertise of relevant disciplines. Through such interdisciplinary cooperation, we are beginning to see gradual improvements in our success at helping people to stop smoking for good.

This kind of cooperation involves not only multiple disciplines but also multiple levels of analysis (see Figure 2.1). At the *intrapersonal* level, for example, the focus is on the individual—his or her genetic background, constitution, developmental experiences, personality characteristics, and so forth. At this level we are concerned with three types of issues: (1) examining factors relevant to assessing predisposition for behavior-related health problems, such as biological dependency (in the case of substance use/abuse), family history of hypertension or obesity,

Figure 2.1
Health Enhancement Planning Model

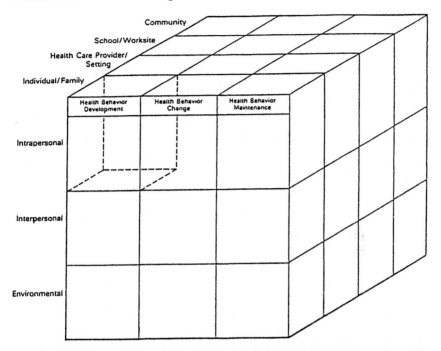

and the ability to successfully cope with life's daily challenges (e.g., self-efficacy measures); (2) developing behavior change strategies to address these problems; and (3) predicting the outcomes of such strategies.

The *interpersonal* level involves all of the social, family, and occupation-related relationships of the individual and how such relationships may enhance or inhibit health behavior development, change, and/or maintenance. Social support, peer pressure, and the family environment are powerful reinforcers of behavior throughout the life cycle. Such socio-cultural influences must be considered as potential agents of change as we come to better understand and define their parameters.

Finally, *environmental* factors, including characteristics of the physical setting as well as legal and policy issues, are also potent determinants of health behaviors. Access to exercise facilities, health assessment procedures, or cigarette machines; the availability of "prudent diet" menus and information at school or worksite cafeterias; the ambient air quality, noise level, and lighting of work and home; the "corporate culture"; and statutory regulations concerning smoking, seat belts, and bicycle helmets all influence health behavior and, presumably, health outcomes (Weiss 1983).

It has been argued, in fact, that in the absence of environmental changes, the likelihood of *maintaining* individual health behavior change is quite low (Brownell, Marlatt, Lichtenstein, and Wilson 1986). Thus, programs that focus on the intrapersonal and interpersonal levels without considering concomitant environmental modification are unlikely to achieve the desired long-term effects.

If this were not sufficiently complex, our model must also differentiate among the processes of health behavior *development* (e.g., brushing teeth, smoking prevention, developing prudent dietary habits), health behavior *change* (shifting from one set of behaviors to another), and health behavior *maintenance* (adherence/preventing relapse). Technical approaches to achieving designated objectives in each area may be quite different. Also, differences in populations may require strategies tailored to the needs of particular groups.

By extending the model into this third dimension, we can recognize the "person-situation" interactions that have special meaning for health behavior. In Figure 2.1, patient-provider, student-school, employee-worksite, and individual-family categories provide examples of person-environment interactions offering potentially useful opportunities for successful health behavior manipulations.

Basic principles predict that certain behaviors will occur, and having once occurred, will occur again and again. Classical conditioning and operant learning theory are rich sources of information about stimulus-response relationships. These relationships are mediated by gradients of reinforcement, stimulus control, generalization/discrimination, modeling, contingency management, excitation/inhibition, motivation, and so forth.

Although these represent some of the components of behavior modification, several other behavioral principles are also considered important in health behavior change. Cognitive restructuring (Meichenbaum 1977) involves the reappraisal of thoughts and perceptions regarding behavior and social relationships. Social support and social integration are concerned with the quality and quantity of our relationship with others. Enhancing quality of life has become an important concept in medical decisionmaking and personal choices about health, including adherence to medical regimens. Behavioral intervention strategies rely heavily on individual self-regulation and self-evaluation. Self-regulation processes reflect personal beliefs, self-appraisals, internal standards of conduct, and perceptions of the external environment. Beliefs involve personal values and the salience of health information for the individual. Self-evaluation, in contrast, concerns the assessment of personal skills and capabilities as they relate to one's beliefs, values, and standards.

The concepts of self-efficacy and social modeling (Bandura 1986) deserve special mention as we consider generic principles of health behavior change. Effective change efforts appear to be highly related to self-perception, coping skills, and the availability of salient role models. As one's perception of oneself becomes increasingly consistent with valued social norms, as coping repertoires expand in size and variety, and as identification with positive models takes place, the likelihood of successful health behavior development, change, and maintenance is correspondingly enhanced. One must consider how to maximize these dimensions in planning targeted interventions.

Our research experiences in the fields of learning and behavior modification have generated a "technology" of behavior change and maintenance at the clinical and small group level. This technology has been expanded to the public health domain through concepts of social marketing (LeFebvre, Harden, Rakowski, Lasater, and Carleton 1987), communication (Winett, 1987); Solomon and Maccoby 1984), community organization (e.g., Rogers and Kincaid 1981), and social learning (Bandura 1986). Theoretical models designed to influence the lifestyle behaviors of populations (e.g., communities) are presently being tested in several community risk-reduction programs throughout the United States and Europe.

To review these principles in detail is beyond the scope and intent of this chapter. However, they represent the basic theoretical and experimental underpinnings for clinical and public health interventions currently being used to effect behavior change in individuals, selected groups, and populations.

Understanding how such principles apply to the health problems of the developing, as well as the "developed," world is one of the challenges facing us. If the health problems of the developing world turn out to resemble those of western countries, we may expect to see a significant increase in cardiovascular and neoplastic diseases and stroke, accompanied by an increased incidence of hypertension, particularly in the more urbanized segment of the population. The opportunity for considering truly preventive strategies, such as attempting to reverse the smoking and dietary patterns in this population, is unquestionably tempting. Unfortunately, the current health problems of the developing world are already overtaxing limited national expenditures, and problems associated with the newly emerging chronic diseases will have to wait until more pressing issues are brought under control.[1] These include clean air and water, sanitation and waste disposal, control of infectious disease vectors, immunization, maternal and child health, and preventable injuries—health problems very similar to those faced by the now-industrialized countries 100 to 200 years ago. The geopolitical and environmental conditions of today's Third World countries—climate, population density, geography, inadequate raw material and industrial base, political systems—combine to perpetuate a "vicious cycle" subsistence economy. If it is not possible to gather sufficient resources to improve the health of a population, that population cannot produce more than what is required for bare sustenance. The resources necessary to improve public health therefore cannot be provided. Given limited resources, improvements in the health status of a population are unlikely to come from the more expensive "curative" side of health care technology.

Fortunately, in most cases these problems can be addressed by relatively inexpensive and uncomplicated interventions. However, the problems of presenting such interventions to a population in a socially and culturally acceptable form—that is, getting people to adopt the necessary changes as "their own" and build the infrastructure necessary to sustain these changes—requires collaborative efforts from many disciplines integrated within a common conceptual framework. For example, the epidemiologist studies patterns of disease incidence and prevalence within a given environment. The results of epidemiological research provide extremely valuable clues to sources of the health problem. The anthropologist and sociologist survey and explore cultural and social contexts, while the psychologist attempts to determine both objective and perceptual issues from the standpoint of the individual. The biologist, physician, physiologist, and geneticist each work at different levels of analysis to improve our understanding of a given health problem. Thus, the contribution of each member of a multidisciplinary team provides an important addition to the mosaic.

We need to incorporate what we have learned from clinical and public health approaches to lifestyle modification (e.g., worksite and community risk reduction programs) into an integrated model that can be adapted to the health concerns of the developing world. Combining the more sophisticated tools of behavioral analysis and modifications—social marketing, communication theory, social modeling, self-efficacy theory, cognitive-behavioral restructuring, self-management strategies—with concepts like social support, social networks, and enhancement of quality of life, we can approach each of the concerns at the intrapersonal, interpersonal, and environmental levels, devising strategies relevant to health behavior development, change, and maintenance. Community organizations, cultural and social networks, "barefoot doctors," traditional healers and other indigenous resources are potential agents for facilitating behavior change within a given cultural milieu.

The media, for example, has proven to be a particularly effective agent of change in western societies when employed in the context of a multifaceted program of behavior change. This medium must be adapted and pilot-tested in representative developing world populations. Restricted access to electronic media, illiteracy rates, and problems of geographical distribution pose special challenges to communication theory experts as they work to develop strategies that will reach (and have meaning for) these populations.

In considering the major health problems of the developing world, one is struck by the simple and straightforward quality of the diagnostic and treatment skills required. Yet the health care system has failed to establish universally effective programs of oral rehydration therapy (ORT), malaria control and eradication, immunization, potable water, and sanitation/waste disposal. Malnutrition, respiratory diseases, and diarrheal diseases form a "synergistic triad" that, along with malaria, is responsible for millions of deaths of children under five years of age.

In addition to these issues, family planning and adequate infant nutrition are appropriate candidates for behavioral intervention. Social and cultural values in many developing world settings support large families. Attitudes about fertility and virility also pose formidable barriers to change. However, in Asia, children born within one year of previous siblings are two to four times more likely to die compared to those who are born at least three years after the last birth (Winikoff and Brown 1980). Infant nutritional patterns (breast-feeding), age at weaning, contraceptive availability and use, availability of clean water, and adequate sanitation are among the health behavior issues pertinent to child survival.

Health beliefs, often culturally defined, play an important role in the health behavior of a given population. Understanding the nature and origin of such beliefs often provides clues to the most effective and culturally appropriate change agent. For example, health beliefs concerning the relationship of child spacing to likelihood of survival may determine the mother's willingness to modify her behavior. Infant nutrition practices have shifted from breast-feeding to bottle-feeding, particularly in urbanized areas (Meldrum and D. Dominico 1982). This both increases the risk of contracting waterborne diarrheal diseases and deprives the child of the extra immunity provided by breast milk. Bottle-feeding also eliminates the period of decreased fertility for women that comes with lactation.

Successful efforts to reverse these trends or to regain the protective elements of earlier practices will require behavioral and social science research programs directed toward identifying existing belief and incentive systems and designing strategies to encourage the adoption (or readoption) of health-protective behaviors. Several routes for effecting such changes in community health behavior should be considered. Although expert multidisciplinary teams of foreign scientists and health planners can be brought in to test the short-term efficacy of adapted strategies, longer-range objectives should include the development of indigenous infrastructure necessary to continue and extend such work.

Organizing curricula for existing health-related training facilities (e.g., medical schools, schools of nursing); establishing postgraduate training programs for practitioners (including traditional healers); encouraging collaborative activities between host country biomedical and behavioral science disciplines; providing scholarships for young scientists and practitioners from the developed world to engage in research projects in developing countries; and establishing training fellowships for host country personnel to participate in ongoing community, school, and worksite risk reduction programs are all potential avenues of technology transfer and application.

In terms of actual program development, the multidisciplinary behavioral medicine team should be involved at all stages of the design, implementation, and evaluation of health intervention programs. We must trace the cultural, social, and behavioral routes through which infectious diseases are transmitted, as well as tracing the biological mechanisms involved. To reduce parasitic diseases, for example, we must understand exposure patterns. This may involve studying culturally defined excretory and waste management behavior, traditional beliefs concerning disease etiology, infant care and feeding practices, personal protective behavior against biting insects, ritual bathing patterns, and so forth. Environmental hygienists, anthropologists, epidemiologists, psychologists, economists, and health educators, as well as physicians, parasitologists, and biologists, could all provide meaningful input into such a program.

The considerable experience we have accrued in designing and implementing health-related behavioral interventions for the developed world can be put to good use in dealing with Third World health issues. However, such interventions must be tailored to acknowledged health objectives in the context of appropriate cultural, social, and economic parameters if meaningful and long-lasting consequences are to accrue to the society as a whole. Problems such as these cannot be approached in a piecemeal fashion.

As has been the case in industrialized nations, the collective knowledge and skills of many disciplines are required to understand the complexities of health issues in the developing world. The skills and knowledge already exist. The task before us is to integrate them through truly collaborative efforts. Effective collaboration will enable us to generate the multidimensional approaches necessary to address simultaneously multifactorial health problems on all relevant levels.

NOTE

1. One contribution that could be considered on an environmental level, however, would be to halt the export of domestic tobacco and the associated marketing strategies to developing countries.

REFERENCES

Bandura, A. 1986. *Social Foundations of Thought and Action: A Social Cognitive Theory.* Englewood Cliffs, N.J.: Prentice Hall.

Belloc, N., and L. Breslow. 1972. Relationship of Physical Health Status and Health Practices. *Preventive Medicine* 1:409–21.

Brownell, K. D., G. A. Marlatt, E. Lichtenstein, and G. T. Wilson. 1986. Understanding and Preventing Relapse. *American Psychologist* 41:765–82.

Kannel, W. B., T. R. Dawber, A. Kagan, N. Revotski, and J. Stokes. 1961. Factors of Risk in the Development of Coronary Heart Disease: Six-Year Follow-Up Experience. *Annals of Internal Medicine* 55:33–50.

Lalonde, M. 1974. *A New Perspective on the Health of Canadians.* Ottawa: Ministry of National Health and Welfare.

LeFebvre, R. C., E. A. Harden, W. Rakowski, T. M. Lasater, and R. A. Carleton. 1987. Characteristics of Participants in Community Health Promotion Programs: Four-Year Results. *American Journal of Public Health* 77:10:1342–44.

Meichenbaum, D. 1977. *Cognitive Behavior Modification: An Integrative Framework.* New York: Plenum.

Meldrum, B., and C. DiDominico. 1982. Production and Reproduction. Women and Breastfeeding: Some Nigerian Examples. *Social Science and Medicine* 16:1247.

Rogers, E. M., and D. C. Kincaid. 1981. *Communication Networks: Toward a New Paradigm for Research.* New York: Free Press.

Schwartz, G. E., and S. M. Weiss. 1978. Behavioral Medicine Revisited: An Amended Definition. *Journal of Behavioral Medicine* 1:3:249–51.

Solomon, D. S., and N. Maccoby. 1984. Communications as a Model for Health Enhancement. In *Behavioral Health: A Handbook for Health Enhancement and Disease Prevention.* J. D. Matarazzo, S. M. Weiss, J. A. Herd, N. E. Miller, and S. M. Weiss, eds. New York: Wiley.

Weiss, S. M. 1982. Health Psychology: The Time Is Now. *Health Psychology* 1:1:4–13.

———. 1983. Health and Illness: The Behavioral Medicine Perspective. In *Emotions in Health and Illness.* L. S. Zegans, L. Temoshok, and C. VanDyke, eds. New York: Academic Press.

Winett, R. A., K. O. Kramer, W. B. Walker, S. W. Malone, and M. K. Lane. 1987. Effective Consumer Information Interventions: Concept, Design, and Impacts Using Field Experiments. In *Telecommunications and Demand Modeling: An Integrative Review.* A. deFontenay, D. Sibley, and M. Shugard, eds. Amsterdam: North Holland.

Winikoff, B., and G. Brown. 1980. Nutrition, Population and Health: Theoretical and Practical Issues. *Social Science and Medicine* 14C:171–76.

3

Research Possibilities on Facilitating the Health Care Transition

DAVID MECHANIC

It may be useful to think of the health care transition in two stages. In the initial stage, educational and public health measures are directed at infectious and communicable disease that can be reduced by prudent measures to insure a safe source of water, appropriate management of waste products, adequate sanitation, and the application of preventive health care.[1] Since these approaches are relatively focused and effective, impressive advances can occur relatively quickly. These advances are indexed by sharp reductions in infant, child, and maternal mortality.

The implementation of the first stage usually requires some degree of community mobilization through a set of attitudes we might call "psychological modernity," as well as the rudimentary organization of primary health care that is accessible and oriented to public health practice. Some degree of psychological modernity is necessary to motivate the population to use primary health care facilities, to cooperate in care, and to adhere to advice and instruction. However, the necessary level of modernity and the educational experience that induces it is relatively modest if the system of primary care is economically, physically, and culturally accessible and maintains a preventive orientation with aggressive community outreach. A strong psychological modernity orientation can overcome an inefficiently organized primary care system, but a well-organized system of care can have impressive results even in highly traditional contexts.

The second stage of the health transition encompasses a broader range of the life cycle, a multiplicity of diseases with varying causes, and less proven social and technological interventions. It poses more difficult challenges. Here the goal is to add increments of health and increased longevity at various points in the life cycle, including old age. Possible instruments for achieving this goal are both varied and more uncertain. Moreover, the interventions themselves—for example, those related to diet, work and environmental risks, accidents, and high risk behaviors—have much broader economic implications than those characteristic of the earlier stage. At any given level of economic development, progress in the second stage is likely to depend in a much deeper sense on the degree of psychological modernity and the quality of social organization.

Persons who have developed attitudes of psychological modernity in Alex Inkeles's terms, take on "new transformative roles within their societies and in their more immediate social networks." Such persons

adopt different social roles than do their less modern countrymen. They are more active in voluntary organizations and participate more in politics; they practice birth control more regularly and have fewer children as a result; they are quicker to adopt innovative practices in agriculture and are more productive as workers in industry; they keep their children longer in school and encourage them to take up more technical occupations; and, in general, they press more actively for social change. (Inkeles 1983: 26–27)

The single most important factor associated with psychological modernity is formal schooling. Inkeles has argued that much of the effect of formal schooling comes not from curricula but from responses to the structure of the classroom situation itself. Ordered sequences of activities and scheduling, modeling, and other psychosocial processes are examples of classroom structure (Inkeles and Smith 1974: 140–42). A similar argument has been made for the ways in which factory work structures activities and dispositions. The structure of factory work also seems to have an important effect, but one less powerful than schooling.

Schooling is an influential determinant of health in developed as well as developing countries. It has effects that are independent of income and occupation, with which it is also substantially correlated. Schooling is associated with a wide range of psychosocial characteristics, including cognitive complexity, self-concept, active coping, sense of mastery, aggressiveness in seeking information, and conceptual skills in managing information (Mechanic 1989). Persons with more schooling not only have more knowledge, but they also are inclined to continue to acquire knowledge (Feldman 1966). When exposed to new information, they assimilate more than those with less schooling. Spaeth (1976) has suggested that socioeconomic levels can be viewed as indicators of cognitive complexity. Children exposed to better educated models, whether parents or teachers, learn to cope more actively with complex situations.

The schooling variable provides a possible window into the arena for interventions, but it also has some limitations. First, schooling is an enabling factor that makes a variety of outcomes more possible. However, the consequences of schooling are dependent on values that may be exogenous. In the developing countries, schooling is associated with increased female autonomy, control of fertility, and a higher quality of prenatal and infant care. In modern societies, the fact that female autonomy may be associated with a variety of increased health risks, such as smoking or use of alcohol and drugs, suggests the complexity of causal pathways. Second, as experience in modern nations illustrates, getting children to school does not necessarily mean they will find there cultures that promote values of academic achievement, skill acquisition, or positive health behavior. Schooling is a measure of exposure, but depending on context, it remains something of a "black box." Third, school entry, progression, and attrition are complex social selection processes that may result in our attributing more influence to the context of schooling than to the capacities, personal characteristics, and values of families that persist in keeping children in school despite economic and other costs.

Schooling promotes health enhancement because it potentially (1) teaches skills that facilitate the acquisition and manipulation of health knowledge and (2) induces psychological modernity. It is the culture of the kinship group and community, however, that propels these orientations in one or another direction. As one considers varying health risks throughout the life span, it becomes clear that much of the relevant behavior is shaped by norms and routine activities that may inadvertently contribute to or damage health. Only very little health-relevant behavior is governed by health-conscious motives. Health is a derivative of the everyday structure of routines, activities, and socioeconomic circumstances.

Thus, promoting health in the second stage of the health transition is much more difficult than in the first stage, because it is an exercise in changing culture. The challenge is to introduce modern attitudes with minimal disruption of the web of relationships, loyalties, and dependencies that exist in a given cultural setting. Rapid modernization and technical change often result in generational conflict, disruption of traditional culture, and high levels of anomie and alienation. These effects contribute to personal pathology and violence. As populations move from rural to urban centers in search of new opportunities, and as they confront the realities of urban poverty and unemployment, they may have few replacements for the traditional web of helping relationships and patterns of sustenance they left behind.

A health-enhancing environment must deal not only with the issues of economic subsistence but also with the broader context of cultural integrity, group structure, and personal meanings. It must insure enough cultural integrity to provide a solid basis for family planning and childhood socialization, a positive orientation to education, and an ethic that gives work and productivity a meaningful place in the group's value structure. This is unlikely unless each family feels it has a stake in the future through its own efforts or those of its children.

It is unclear how we can induce social change and modify cultural configurations without causing major disruptions. If the initial cultural configuration is strong and adapts well to modern development, it can provide the basis for using knowledge to enhance child development, nutrition, safety, and other behavior patterns consistent with health.

TARGETS FOR INTERVENTION

In many areas of the world, efforts to promote the first stage of the health transition are still rudimentary. This is a result of extreme poverty, poor access to basic public health and preventive health care services, and highly traditional cultures that erect major barriers to female education and participation outside the household. When care is poorly organized and inaccessible, greater personal initiative is required to secure it. In contrast, an aggressive outreach effort that works within the context of existing cultural configurations can compensate for cultural and educational impediments to care.

Cultural patterns that inhibit female education and participation outside the household, and that discriminate against females with respect to nutrition, medical care, and schooling, are formidable barriers. These patterns are typically quite tenacious and resistant to change techniques outside the context of significant economic development and modernization. We do not know a great deal about how to effectively introduce modern medical and fertility planning in these contexts. Nor do we understand what approaches are most persuasive when fertility control poses challenges to important principles of traditional culture. I suspect this is one of the reasons education is such a powerful proxy for modernization. Schooling provides the opportunity to offer alternatives to the traditional culture as well as induce some of the habits and skills essential for participation in a modern economy.

In contexts where there is resistance to education, either for religious or cultural reasons or because schooling interferes with economic activity, individual interventions have limited promise. The use of respected, credible face-to-face influence has more potential than more impersonal forms of communication, but in either case it would be foolish to expect too much. One begins by seeking change in areas that pose the least challenge to core cultural ideas, and one builds in iterative steps to encompass more central spheres of health-relevant activity. Trust is essential, and it is strategic to begin with areas of intervention that yield visible and valued outcomes that clearly can be attributed to the intervention.

The behavioral orientations that intervene between macro-forces and specific behaviors conducive to health—attitudes and attributions, cognitive capacities, and effectiveness in acquiring and using information—are affected by many sociocultural and situational factors other than education. In theory, these are amenable to direct intervention. However, existing health behavior theories are not particularly powerful tools for shaping organized programs for changing health-relevant behavior. A wide variety of factors have been identified that make individuals more or less susceptible to the adoption of innovations in particular instances, but the theories are not specific enough to provide a clear guide to action (Rogers and Shoemaker 1971). If one goal is to change cultural attributions and understandings that impede positive health action, then existing evidence roughly suggests that we have two general tasks. First, we have to induce motivation for change by convincing individuals that certain behaviors are damaging to valued goals and that change would bring significant benefits. Second, we have to convey how the desired behavior can be implemented in a comfortable way without extensive costs in time, money, or erosion of cherished values.

If we take these guidelines seriously, we may be able to order communities along a spectrum of amenability to change. In some instances, we face enormous difficulty in inducing the necessary motivation because of religious and other cultural constraints. In other instances, the motivation is more or less present and the challenge is to devise an operational phase that assists communities in implementing desired behaviors. Similarly, even in communities where motivation appears low, it may be possible to target subgroups in the population who have greater readiness for change and who might over time become effective change agents.

QUESTIONS AND NEEDED RESEARCH

How susceptible are societies to changes in their underlying attitudes? I know of no evidence that would lead us to anticipate that core values can be modified without fundamental socioeconomic changes, but I doubt that this is a particularly useful way to think about the challenge. Most societies place a reasonable value on health irrespective of their particular core values, and we would have to define our health objectives quite specifically to assess conflicts between core values and these objectives. We probably know more about conflicts in fertility control than in any other area, but family planning experiences may not be particularly representative. While fertility control is associated with many crucial issues affecting health and development, it also involves strong competing perceptions of the economic and social implications of fe-cundity. In contrast, maternal survival, infant survival, and child health are valued to a high degree in all cultures. Impediments are typically associated more with organizational and economic barriers than with value conflict. Obviously, how a service is defined and delivered may result in more or less resistance depending on the compatibility of the service configuration with the values of the group. But in any specific instance, understanding values provides opportunities for presenting the service in an acceptable way. The extent to which such special efforts are necessary depends on the psychological modernity of the clients served.

We might conceive of fulfillment of a particular health objective as an endpoint on a continuum involving a variety of barriers. Such barriers may involve tangible costs, such as money, time, physical distance, or effort and discomfort; or social costs, such as embarrassment, stigma, or social distance. Such barriers might be modified either by reconcep-tualizing how services are organized and provided (such as through improved physical access, outreach, or increased sensitivity to cultural concerns) or by inducing among individuals the confidence and skills to overcome roadblocks to appropriate care. While the latter approach might seem preferable, the former is probably more readily achieved.

But even with the organizational approach there is need for a clear understanding of how notions of health and illness are constructed in varying cultural circumstances, how attributions are made about cause and threat, and how meanings are assigned. This requires some local anthropology to assess how misunderstanding can best be avoided, how behavioral modifications might best be achieved, and what types of indigenous networks might be mobilized to accomplish health objectives.

We still do not know how to address populations that lack substantial intrinsic motivation to pursue health objectives because of major conflicts with other culturally valued goals. I once was the guest of a Bedouin who had fathered 26 children and was negotiating for an additional wife to continue to add to his family. Local clinicians indicated that several of his children had a "failure to thrive" syndrome resulting from un-dernutrition. Yet the presence of foreign guests prompted the presen-tation of a meal that had the appearance of affluence.

This small example conveys some of the difficulties we must confront. The introduction of incentives might immediately change the priorities. I doubt, however, that we have any incentives that are practical enough to be broadly applied. Instead, we have to think about interventions that promise greater potential for success over two or three generations.

While there may be few viable incentives to change the personal prior-ities of my Bedouin host, it might be somewhat easier to induce him to allow his children to continue in school and, perhaps, outdistance him in terms of psychological modernity. While some of his children had been to school, he viewed schooling as having little value. But with sufficient external incentive he might be persuaded to continue to send his children to school despite his low opinion of education.

We do not know a great deal about external inducers and how large they have to be to achieve varying objectives. It seems evident, however, that our chances for success are much enhanced with collective mobilization of communities around important health targets. One form such mobilization can take is a political process initiated through public policy efforts, as in rural China's voluntary health initiatives that mobilized community public health and preventive efforts. Alternatively, community mobilization may be part of community health education efforts combining outreach, community organization, and identification of indigenous leadership. We have a lot of practical experience in these areas, but we do not know very much about what works and why.

There is danger in becoming too grandiose in our objectives. Throughout the world, there are large populations already motivated to curtail their fertility, to seek early prenatal and child care, and to enhance their life chances. But a large gap remains in most countries between intention and implementation. In countries throughout Africa, Asia, and Latin America, many women who seek to delay pregnancy are not using birth control. The failures are likely to be more in the organization of fertility control efforts than in attitudes. It would serve us well to understand much better than we now do the intervening factors that lead to large gaps between intention and behavior.

Over the long term, the issue is how to encourage the evolution of psychological modernity in a way that minimizes cultural dislocations and personal anomie. One approach is through education: increasing schooling opportunities for boys and girls, making efforts to delay the school leaving age, and working to improve the fit between a better educated labor force and economic opportunities. In many countries throughout the world, impoverished populations are abandoning rural areas to settle in large cities without appreciable economic opportunities. Such dislocations may accelerate processes of modernization, but not without high social and personal costs.

In sum, there are several levels on which the health transition might be addressed. Perhaps the simplest, but one with great potential, is to better understand the barriers that prevent individuals from translating their desire for good health into effective behavior. Such deficiencies may be largely organizational and economic and may require reorganization and redirection of primary health services and family planning. A related, second level is to examine alternative approaches to improve performance in such areas as prenatal and maternal care, child monitoring, and immunization and basic health services. Values concerning the health of mothers and children are sufficiently strong in most cultures to make these populations productive targets. A third level is to examine economic, legal, and other regulatory approaches that induce health motivation. A fourth is to examine possible vehicles for encouraging psychological modernity through education or other means. Attitudes can be extremely important, but attitudes also often change in response to social and technological change. Effective change efforts will require modifications of both material conditions and how individuals assign meanings to their changing environments.

NOTE

1. Preventive health care includes prenatal care, safe childbirth practices, immunization, and appropriate infant nutrition.

REFERENCES

Feldman, J. 1966. *The Dissemination of Health Education.* Chicago: Aldine.
Inkeles, A. 1983. *Exploring Individual Modernity.* New York: Columbia University Press.
Inkeles, A., and D. H. Smith. 1974. *Becoming Modern.* Cambridge, Mass.: Harvard University Press.
Mechanic, D. 1989. Socioeconomic Status and Health: An Examination of Underlying Processes. In *Pathways to Health: The Role of Social Factors.* J. P. Bunker, D. S. Gomby, and B. H. Kehrer, eds. Menlo Park, CA: Henry J. Kaiser Family Foundation.
Rogers, E. M., and F. F. Shoemaker. 1971. *Communication of Innovations: A Cross-Cultural Approach.* New York: Free Press.
Spaeth, J. L. 1976. Cognitive Complexity: A Dimension Underlying the Socioeconomic Achievement Process. In *Schooling and Achievement in American Society.* W. H. Sewell, R. M. Hanser, and D. L. Featherman, eds. New York: Academic Press.

PART II
CASE STUDIES

4

The Rise and Fall of the Cigarette: A Brief History of the Antismoking Movement in the United States

ALLAN M. BRANDT

INTRODUCTION

In the last 25 years, American society has witnessed a revolution in attitudes and behaviors relating to cigarette smoking. When Surgeon General Luther Terry announced at a nationally televised press conference in January 1964 that his official commission on smoking and health had concluded that smoking causes lung cancer and other disease, there were 70 million adult smokers in the United States who consumed some 400 billion cigarettes each year (Surgeon General's Report 1964). By 1989, the percentage of smokers in the United States had fallen from 42 percent to 26 percent. The decline in cigarette smoking is only the most obvious marker of an important historical transformation in attitudes and values about health, disease, and behavioral risks. Half of all living Americans who have ever smoked have now quit. According to the most recent Surgeon General's Report, approximately 750,000 smoking related deaths have been avoided since 1964 because people have quit or not started smoking (Surgeon General's Report 1989). Terry's Surgeon General's Report marked the beginning of a profound redefinition of the cigarette; moreover, it spurred new interests more generally in the relationship of behavior, risk, and health.

Although the decline in cigarette smoking in the United States has been widely noted, the history of this change has gone largely unexplored. Perhaps this is because for many educated Americans the demise of the cigarette seems self-evident. Once the evidence that smoking constituted a serious health risk was mounted, once physicians and the public were appropriately apprised of these risks, the public would obviously stop smoking. But changes in behavior, as medical social science has amply demonstrated, are more difficult and complex than such a simple and rational model would hold, especially when those behaviors are addictive (Leventhal and Cleary 1980). No simple rationalistic model can account for such a significant change on an individual or societal level. And indeed, consumption of cigarettes in the United States continued to rise in the decade following the first Surgeon General's Report in spite of growing awareness of the risks of serious disease.

This chapter will attempt to account for the decline of cigarette smoking in the United States by evaluating a range of historical variables that contributed to this change. There are, of course, some obvious markers: the development of powerful epidemiologic data; the ability to effectively communicate such risks to the public; the role of the federal government in providing authoritative information concerning risk; the organization of a consumer movement with an effective political lobby; a growing recognition on the part of public health advocates of the power of the media in shaping health consciousness. All of these are obvious elements in the shift that we will briefly explore. Nevertheless, it is important to note that even this set of factors cannot adequately explain the transformation in attitudes, values, and behaviors over the last quarter century. For this reason, it will be necessary as well to briefly examine certain aspects of American cultural beliefs about behavior, disease, and health that contributed as well to the change.

Such an analysis is particular and idiosyncratic. It will attempt to examine the specific set of circumstances that led to changes in a specific nation at a specific time. What relevance does the American experience have to our understanding of the health transition in the less developed world? History, of course, is not a fable with a moral spelled out at the end. Nevertheless, the clearer our understanding of the changes that occurred in the United States, the better the possibility of constructing a "usable past." Fully explicating those forces that led to change in one society—as well as those that continue to serve as obstacles—offers us the opportunity to identify socially and culturally specific forces that may be significant in other nations to promote health or prevent disease. In this respect, a fuller analysis of a specific "health transition" in the United States may have implications for health policies in the developing world.

THE RISE OF THE CIGARETTE

Before any consequential campaign to reduce cigarette smoking could be mounted, conclusive evidence of the hazards of smoking had to be demonstrated. However, this process of clearly specifying risk, to "prove" that cigarettes cause disease, was complex. It required both the development of new statistical and quantitative techniques and a re-thinking of the very nature of causal relationships in epidemiology.

As long as there have been cigarettes, there have been concerns about their impact on health. As consumption of mass-produced cigarettes rose dramatically in the early twentieth century, many physicians and social reformers raised questions about their implications for health and morals. By the time of World War I, some 13 states had enacted legislation prohibiting or regulating the sale of cigarettes; anticigarette activists often cited medical and scientific experts in support of such restrictions (Sobel 1978).

Despite these concerns, cigarette consumption continued to increase. In many ways the cigarette seems such a ubiquitous part of American culture that it is difficult to imagine it is really a twentieth-century phenomenon. Per capita consumption rose from 1900 to 1965, as indicated by the following figures:

1900	49
1910	138
1920	611
1930	1,365
1940	1,828
1950	3,322
1960	3,889
1965	4,318

Obviously, a full account of the rise of the cigarette is beyond the scope of this chapter. Developments in agricultural technique, production technology, and industrial organization, as well as such factors as the introduction of the portable match, all contributed to the growth of the tobacco industry (Bennett 1980). The advent of the cigarette marks the convergence of corporate capitalism, technology, mass marketing, and in particular, the impact of advertising (Schudson 1985). These forces signaled new modes of individual and group behavior. With the rise of consumerism, a new behavioral ethic was defined. After the promotion of self-denial and self-discipline in the late nineteenth century—a culture that condemned indulgence in all forms—American were now encouraged to indulge.

As individuals feared the loss of autonomy in an industrial world, cigarette smoking promised individual redemption. The Marlboro man was the first urban-industrial cowboy, a symbol of modernity, autonomy, power, and sexuality. Such advertising pointed away from the product toward the moral and psychological value of the patron (Fox and Lears 1983). Advertising promised consumers well-being and power

(Marchand 1985). Creating demand for relatively undifferentiated, non-essential items was the core of the new consumer culture that the cigarette epitomizes. The tobacco industry boomed, as did state revenues associated with the manufacture and sale of cigarettes. As demand for cigarettes rose, so too did concern about their impact on health.

MODERN EPIDEMIOLOGY AND STATISTICAL INFERENCE

By the late 1920s, researchers began to focus more precisely on the specific consequences of smoking. As early as 1928, in a somewhat primitive epidemiological study, researchers associated heavy smoking with cancer (Lombard and Doering 1928). In addition, surgeons published clinical reports associating cancer in their patients with their smoking habits (Ochsner 1973). In 1931, Frederick L. Hoffman, a well-known statistician for the Prudential Insurance Company, tied smoking to cancer. Hoffman noted the difficulties of conducting epidemiological studies in this area. The basic methodological questions of statistical research; issues of representativeness, sample size, and the construction of control groups all presented researchers with a series of complex problems. Hoffman concluded by calling for the exercise of moderation in all behavior, a truism of Progressive hygiene, suggesting that "extreme moderation in smoking habits would certainly be advisable" (Hoffman 1931).

In 1938, Raymond Pearl, a Johns Hopkins statistician and biometrician, published the first significant statistical analysis of the health impact of smoking. Pearl came to the conclusion that in individuals it was difficult to assess the risks of such behaviors, especially when their impact was not immediate and when there were many intervening variables that also influenced health. Therefore, he concluded, the only precise way to evaluate their effect on health was to employ statistical methods, collecting data on large groups of individuals. Comparing the mortality curves of smokers and nonsmokers, Pearl found that individuals who smoked could expect shorter lives. He offered no explanation as to why this might be so (Pearl 1938).

During the 1920s and 1930s, as the first studies attempting to link cigarettes to cancer were conducted, epidemiology as a field stood at a crossroads. The bacteriological revolution of the late nineteenth and early twentieth century had redirected attention away from the traditional environmental questions that had brought epidemiology to the fore. Questions came to center on the issue of mechanism: identifying causative agents, universally assumed to be microorganisms. Indeed, the notion that disease was actually "caused" by hazards in the environment fell into disrepute as public health officers were compelled to demonstrate Robert Koch's postulates, the fundamental truths of the new germ theory. There were, of course, exceptions to this trend, especially the development of industrial and occupational health. But for the most part these fields were distant from the central concerns of biomedicine and public health. And in fact it is worth noting that the major statistical work of the period came from the fields of population genetics and the actuarial studies of the insurance industry, rather than from the disciplines of public health. Neither Hoffman nor Pearl would have considered themselves epidemiologists.

The municipal laboratory had become the new focus of public health. Even when researchers identified environmental or behavioral risks, they generally focused on the mechanism of disease. The notion of statistical inference was questioned as research centered on the cellular level. In this respect, exposure to a carcinogen was equated with exposure to an infectious organism. Identifying the health risks of a particular behavior like smoking fitted this model poorly. The length of time before the disease developed was protracted (and equated to an "incubation period"); in addition, the large number of intervening variables confounded notions of specific causality. Everyone "exposed" did not get the disease; indeed, most did not. There was also broad cultural discomfort with notions of comparative risk assessment. How dangerous was the cigarette.? How did this danger rate vis-à-vis other risks? Finally, biomedicine offered few persuasive models for understanding systemic and chronic diseases; the anomalies of cigarette smoking did not fit the biomedical model's ideal of specific causality.

Changing patterns of disease, however, forced researchers to search for other models of causality. By the end of World War II, concern about lung cancer had intensified. It seemed to statisticians and physicians to be a striking exception to many other disease patterns of the twentieth century; deaths from lung cancer had risen from 4,000 in 1935 to 11,000 in 1945. By 1960 the number of annual lung cancer deaths would rise to 36,000 (Hammond 1962). Carcinoma of the lung would become by the mid–1980s the most prevalent of all cancers, accounting for more than 140,000 deaths each year. At the turn of the twentieth century the disease was almost unheard of, with fewer than 400 cases recorded in 1900.

There were, of course, many theories to account for this shift. Some observers attributed the rise in cases to better reporting, more sophisticated diagnostic abilities, the widespread use of Xrays, and the ability to make precise pathological analyses. Alternative theories suggested that increasing life expectancy permitted the development of disease that in an earlier era would not have had the chance to wreak its havoc on victims because they would have died earlier from other causes (Little 1961).

But others pointed to one of the most dramatic behavioral changes in the history of American culture, the rise of cigarette smoking. By the late 1940s it was already known that prolonged exposure to certain industrial chemicals and vapors—chromate, nickel carbonyl, and radio-active dusts—could produce lung cancer. Some scientists now suggested that the inhalation of cigarette smoke might have similar effects. This hypothesis led to a series of epidemiological studies of the risk of smoking. These studies, in turn, led to a redefinition of risk epidemiology, and public health.

First published in the 1950s, these investigations were based upon retrospective findings. In other words, individuals with lung cancer were identified in hospitals and interviewed regarding their smoking practices; they were then compared to a similar group who did not smoke. According to the data, cigarette smokers were at far higher risk for the development of lung cancer than were nonsmokers. But critics raised a series of objections to such studies. In particular, it was clear that there were a number of opportunities for bias in the construction of sample and control groups. For example, it was suggested that lung cancer patients were likely, because of the nature of their disease, to exaggerate their smoking habits (Doll and Hill 1952).

Because of some of the methodological problems with retrospective studies, in 1951 two major prospective studies on smoking and cancer were begun. Under the auspices of the British Medical Research Council, Richard Doll and Bradford Hill sent questionnaires on smoking practices to all British physicians. When members of the profession died, Doll and Hill were able to obtain data concerning the cause of their deaths. The results confirmed the earlier findings of the retrospective studies (Doll and Hill 1954, 1956).

A second major prospective study conducted by E. Cuyler Hammond under the auspices of the American Cancer Society came to similar conclusions. Total death rates among smokers were far higher than among nonsmokers. Lung cancer deaths were 3 to 9 times as high among smokers than among nonsmokers; 5 to 16 times as high among heavy smokers. Among those who smoked two or more packs a day, the death rates were 2.25 times as high as for men who had never smoked. Excess mortality was even higher for coronary artery disease than for lung cancer; rates for smokers exceeded those for nonsmokers by 70 percent. Hammond found that quitting reduced risk; a heavy smoker himself, he now quit (Hammond and Horn 1958a, 1986b). By 1960, a range of epidemiological studies all had arrived at consistent findings: Cigarette smoking significantly contributed to lung cancer and coronary artery disease (Cornfield 1959).

These epidemiological studies introduced the idea of large sample surveys. They centered attention on the definition of comparative risk and excess mortality. Implicit in such studies was a critique of the whole notion of specific causality; these researchers recognized that there were literally hundreds of variables affecting the incidence of disease. Therefore, they sought to design studies that included many individuals and thereby would be controlled except for a single variable—in this case, cigarette smoking.

This type of research touched off an important debate within the scientific community about the nature of causality, proof, and risk. At stake were the very epistemological foundations of scientific knowledge: How do we know what we know? What is the reliability of causal inference from statistical data? Those committed to hereditarian, genetic views of cancer, for example, found fault with this epidemiologic approach that centered attention on behavioral effects (Fisher 1957).

At the basis of the epidemiological argument was the clear limitation of laboratory experimentation for making determinations about probability and risk. The debate about smoking and health revealed an intraprofessional battle between epidemiology and lab science, their values, assumptions, and expectations. Moreover, the debate revealed a deeper discomfort with statistical logic and quantitative methods in biomedicine, a trend that persists today (Feistein 1967). Before any successful anticigarette campaign could be waged, the legitimacy of epidemiological data for generating health policy would have to be established.

FROM EPIDEMIOLOGY TO PUBLIC POLICY

Knowledge of the risks of smoking—which continued to accrue throughout the 1950s—did not immediately lead to the formulation of public policy. And, indeed, there was considerable debate about the implications of these findings for public health authorities. What was the appropriate role of the state vis-à-vis the risks of cigarette smoking? Should the government play a role in educating its citizens about the hazards of smoking? Recognizing the gravity of the hazard, should the government take steps to regulate the sale of cigarettes more aggressively or to restrict their use? These questions, of course, were complicated by the nature of the behavior itself. No one need be exposed to the hazards of smoking unless they so chose; the "voluntary" nature of the risks, it was argued, militated against any governmental intervention.

The first step the federal government finally took—haltingly—in 1962 was to sponsor a commission to study the evidence that cigarettes were harmful. In some respects this was a curious way to proceed, given the quality of the evidence that already existed. But the creation of the Surgeon General's Advisory Committee on Smoking and Health revealed the political aspects of the debate (Fritschler 1969). First, powerful economic interests repeatedly called the epidemiological findings into question, suggesting that the relationship of cigarettes to disease was "merely statistical" and that no clear and objective findings confirmed these risks "in the laboratory" (Terry 1983). The industry responded to the epidemiological data with advertising campaigns that assured their brands were safe, as well as by the introduction of filter cigarettes with expansive claims for health and safety (Whiteside 1971). Second, there was no single, authoritative "reading" of the evidence that had been mounted. Those forces in the public health establishment, especially the voluntary health agencies, realized that the findings linking cigarettes to disease had to be legitimated in the medical and scientific communities, as well as among the public (Wagner 1971).

The Advisory Committee, appointed in July 1962, explicitly avoided all questions of social policy; their charge was to determine whether or not smoking caused disease. But they conducted no new research. The committee reviewed some 7,000 publications including 3,000 research reports published since 1950. They sought to arrive at a clinical judgment on smoking. As one public health official explained, "What do we (that is, the Surgeon General of the United States Public Health Service) advise our Patient, the American Public, about smoking?" (Surgeon General's Advisory Committee Papers 1964). Implicit in this question was a particular model of public health and the role of the state.

Despite the fact that it offered no new data, the Report nevertheless made a fundamental contribution to the study of causal inference in epidemiological studies. What did it mean to say, for example, that cigarettes *caused* lung cancer? How should cause be distinguished from "associated with" "a factor" or "determinant"? Members of the committee realized the complexity of saying simply that smoking causes cancer. Many individuals could smoke heavily throughout their lives and apparently suffer no adverse consequences; "cause" implied a single process in which A, by necessity, would lead to B. Therefore, they acknowledged the complexity:

It should be said at once that no member of this Committee used the word "cause" in an absolute sense in the area of this study. Although various disciplines and fields of scientific knowledge were represented among the membership, all members shared a common conception of the multiple etiology of biological processes. No member was so naive as to insist upon mono-etiology in pathological processes or in vital phenomena. (Surgeon General's Report 1964)

Yet their conviction was clear: Smoking presented a tremendous risk to health. The committee developed a set of criteria for evaluating causal relationships that has been widely applied since that time. Causal evidence had to be (1) consistent, (2) strong, (3) specific, (4), supportive of appropriate temporal relationships, and (5) coherent (Lilienfeld 1983). At the press conference announcing the committee's findings, Terry was asked whether he would now recommend to a patient to stop smoking. His answer was an unequivocal "yes."

The Report served the political functions on which it was predicated. It provided power and legitimacy to the epidemiologic findings; indeed, the Report was of fundamental importance in raising the stature of epidemiology as a discipline. It made clear that the government would accept broader responsibilities for the determination of risks and public education for disease prevention. The ability of self-interested parties such as the tobacco industry to disparage the findings was now delimited. With the first Surgeon General's Report, the battle against the cigarette was joined; less obvious was how the government would utilize this document in setting a public health agenda.

THE TOBACCO WARS

In retrospect, the immediate public and political response to the Surgeon General's Report appears strikingly naive. Newspapers reporting the findings speculated that the tobacco industry would wither away. The presumption was widely held that smokers—now apprised of the risks—would quickly quit. In Congress, such ideas influenced legislators, who in 1965 passed the Federal Cigarette Labelling and Advertising Act. The legislation established a National Clearinghouse on Smoking and Health to encourage health education about the dangers of smoking. In addition it required that all packs of cigarettes carry a warning: "Caution: Cigarette Smoking May be Hazardous to Your Health." Given that the Surgeon General had found that smoking causes lung cancer, the warning was remarkably weak, indicating the effectiveness of the tobacco lobby on Capitol Hill. It further reflected the relative lack of experience most legislators had with scientific findings. At the hearings concerning this legislation, tobacco spokesmen challenged the findings of the Surgeon General. By treating all perspectives as those of "interested" parties to be brokered in the political process, members of Congress sought compromise. Moreover, the powerful economic interests, especially of tobacco-growing states, acted forcefully to moderate any regulatory initiatives (Whelan 1984). Nevertheless, as scientific studies collected in subsequent Surgeon General's reports continued to indict the cigarette as a major cause of serious disease, Congress took additional action. In 1971, the label was changed to "Warning: The Surgeon General Has Determined That Cigarette Smoking Is Dangerous to Your Health." And in 1985, four rotating labels were mandated (Iglehart 1984, 1986).

Increasingly, the battle over the nature of the risks of smoking would be waged in the media. Luther Terry's effective control of the media, for example, greatly contributed to the success of his committee. First, Terry had appointed a commission of elite scientists and clinicians to study the issue of smoking and health; he successfully obviated any easy dismissal of the Report by requiring the none of its members had previously expressed positions on the dangers of the cigarette (Terry 1983). Second, he invited the tobacco industry to review a list of prospective committee members and reject anyone they desired. This made it impossible for the industry to easily discredit the report. The "secret" meetings of the committee generated widespread speculation in the press during the 18 months of deliberations. This interest culminated in the nationally televised press conference of January 1964. Sunday newspapers throughout the country reported the story on front pages.

In this respect, it is worth contrasting the powerful impact of Terry's Report with the activities of his immediate predecessor, Leroy Burney. In 1957 and 1959, Surgeon General Burney had issued statements concerning the risks of cigarette smoking and the growing evidence that they cause lung cancer. In addition to press releases from his office, Burney sent letters to the *Journal of the American Medical Association* (*JAMA*) announcing his findings (Burney 1959). Burney's letters to *JAMA* were based on an essential premise of public health in twentieth-century American life in which clear lines had been drawn between the spheres of public health and clinical medicine. If a Surgeon General wished to inform the public of important information regarding health—so this premise held—he could do so by communicating with their personal physicians. Thus, a letter to *JAMA* from the Surgeon General constituted a "public announcement."

By 1964, in the aftermath of televised presidential debates, a presidential assassination, and a growing war in East Asia, all powerfully portrayed through the electronic media, the expanding role and possibilities of exploiting media for a range of purposes including public health education was increasingly recognized. Terry's Report and the nationally televised press conference made the Surgeon General, for the first time, into a public figure with access to the media. It gave the office a new meaning and authority, which subsequent Surgeon's General would augment. Indeed, the Surgeon General's principal role—given that the office has little funding or authority to initiate programs—is to speak effectively through the media.

In the struggle concerning the meaning of the cigarette, control of the media was bitterly contested. The tobacco industry had considerable resources to expend in this fight, attempting to allay the growing concerns about the impact of smoking on health. For example, advertisements continued to suggest that smokers were youthful, healthy, attractive, and sexually seductive. Although the Federal Trade Commission took action to demand a higher level of accountability from the industry, regulations were weak and difficult to enforce. The antitobacco forces thus pursued other strategies. A young consumer lawyer, John Banzhaf III, decided to attempt to get the Federal Communications Commission to apply the Fairness Doctrine (for equal air time) to cigarette advertising. He formed the group ASH (Action on Smoking and Health) and after a court struggle, forced the national networks to air antismoking spots in prime time. Anticigarette ads got approximately $40 million of free air time. These public service announcements apparently did have an impact; per capita consumption fell from 4,197 in 1966 to 3,969 in 1970 (Warner 1981). Given the success of this anticigarette media blitz, the industry now acquiesced to a legislative ban on broadcast advertising, thus averting the Fairness Doctrine (Whelan 1984).

Congressional antismoking policy thus proved to be decidedly limited. Modest funding for public education, labeling of packages, and banning broadcast advertising constituted the entire federal program to reduce smoking. Significantly, tobacco subsidies were maintained, placing the government in the ambiguous position of working to limit cigarette smoking while simultaneously contributing to the growth of tobacco. The limits of the federal program revealed the ongoing power of the tobacco lobby and the economic interests that it represents (Sapolsky 1980).

TRANSFORMING THE "MEANING" OF CIGARETTE SMOKING

Further research findings about the nature of the risks of cigarette smoking served to tip the balance in favor of antismoking forces during the last decade. Despite considerable gains in stigmatizing the cigarette, the antismoking forces had, by the late 1970s, foundered on a traditional American libertarian ethic: "It's my body and I'll do with it as I please." In keeping with this powerful cultural ideal, further governmental interference relating to smoking was seen as constituting unjustifiable intrusions into individual decisions, a position heartily endorsed by the Tobacco Institute. It was one thing for the government to inform the public about the dangers of smoking; it was quite another to actually take action to restrict or ban the behavior.

For this reason, scientific studies of the impact of "sidestream" smoke took on special significance. Now, with the publication of studies that demonstrated the risks of exposure to other peoples' cigarette smoke—in particular, a higher risk of lung cancer—the antismoking movement was reinvigorated on the basis of a powerful communitarian ethic: "Do with your own body whatever you like, but you may not expose others to risks that that do not agree to take on themselves." As epidemiologist Michael J. Martin explained, "Many people are willing to take on risk, even an enormous risk, themselves. But few are willing to tolerate even a small risk imposed on them" (Business Week 1987). With the imprimatur of a new Surgeon General's Report (1986), the data on "involuntary" smoking led to remarkable changes in the effectiveness of efforts to restrict smoking in public places (Fielding and Phenow 1988). By mid–1988, 320 local communities had adopted laws restricting smoking in public places, up from 90 to 1985 (Surgeon General's Report 1989).

Another Surgeon General's Report (1988) also called into question the voluntariness of cigarette smoking, now for the smoker. By documenting the addictive qualities of cigarette smoking, the notion of an individual voluntarily deciding to smoke was further undermined. Not surprisingly, the tobacco industry challenged these findings. Walker Merryman, a spokesman for the industry's Tobacco Institute, offered a socially elastic definition of addiction: "I've not heard of anyone holding up a liquor store or mugging an old lady to get the money to buy cigarettes" (Wall Street Journal 1988). Nevertheless, the recognition that cigarette smoking subjects individuals to well-recognized biological processes of transient mood alteration, tolerance, and withdrawal led increasingly to the inclusion of nicotine addiction as one more aspect of substance abuse, a deviant behavior (Henningfield 1984). Moreover, the growing recognition of the difficulty of quitting undercut the notion that smoking was simply a matter of choice.

Studies of the risks of sidestream smoke and the addictive nature of cigarettes were pushed by a growing antismoking coalition that included physicians, public health experts, and aggressive consumer activists. This, of course, is not to question the scientific validity of such studies, but rather to indicate the significance of the relationship between authoritative science and its social and political impacts. This research agenda further encouraged the ongoing process of delegitimizing cigarette smoking in American culture. The cigarette—the icon of our consumer culture, the symbol of pleasure and power, sexuality and individuality—had become suspect. The smoker would subsequently be redefined, in a process that we continue to see played out—from the independent Marlboro man or liberated Virginia Slim—to a new vision of a weak, irrational, and now addicted individual. The innocuous habit had become the noxious addiction. The cigarette had been redefined in ways that we are just beginning to calculate. It touched off a revolution in American values about personal health and behavior.

Increasingly, Americans have come to accept notions of individual responsibility for the systemic and chronic diseases characteristic of the health transition. Because heart disease, cancer, and other diseases are powerfully influenced by a range of individual behaviors including diet, alcohol consumption, and smoking, a number of analysts have come to emphasize the significance of modifying behaviors to effect health status and, more generally, patterns of disease (Knowles 1977).

Such views have particular appeal in the context of American health culture, which has historically emphasized the significance of an individual's responsibility for disease. Americans, in this respect, have largely come to reject fatalistic explanatory models of disease and its causes. Social values have underscored norms that suggest that individuals can exert fundamental control over their own health through careful and rational avoidance of risks. For example, the popularity of the "Just Say No" campaign against drugs reflects an essentially voluntaristic notion of risk.

As effective as such values may be in serving to define appropriate behaviors, they present an important political and cultural irony. According to this behavioral ethic, those who continue to take risks must be held accountable for the results. In this respect, the emphasis on individual responsibility may deny broader social responsibilities for health and disease. This theme, which has developed increasingly powerful adherents in the last decade, actually misrepresents the history of cigarette smoking in the twentieth century. Smoking is a complex behavior that has reflected deep social, cultural, and economic forces, as well as a powerful biological process of addiction. Simply identifying individual behavior as the primary vehicle of risk negates the fact that behavior itself is, at times, beyond the scope of individual agency. Behavior is shaped by powerful currents—cultural, psychological, as well as biological processes—all not immediately within the control of the individual. Behaviors such as cigarette smoking are sociocultural phenomena, not merely individual, or necessarily rational.

The emphasis on personal responsibility for risk-taking and disease has come at the very moment when cigarette smoking is increasingly stratified on the basis of education, social class, and race. In 1985, 35 percent of blacks smoke compared to 29 percent of whites (Fiore, Novotny, Pierce, Hatziandreu, and Davis 1989). For college graduates the proportion of smokers fell from 28 percent in 1974 to 18 percent in 1985; for those without a college degree the decrease during the same period was from 36 to 34 percent (Pierce, Fiore, Novotny, Hatziandreu, and Davis 1989). In this respect, to emphasize individual accountability is to deny that some groups may be more susceptible to certain behavioral risks, that the behavior itself is not simply a matter of choice.

It would be premature to celebrate the decline in cigarette consumption. Cigarettes continue to exact an enormous toll on health in the United States and, increasingly, throughout the world. According to recently revised figures, 390,000 deaths each year are attributed to cigarette smoking (Washington Post 1989). Smoking is estimated to cause 30 percent of all cancer deaths, 21 percent of all deaths from coronary artery disease, and 82 percent of all deaths from chronic obstructive pulmonary disease. Since 1986, lung cancer has become the leading cause of cancer deaths among American women, surpassing breast cancer, the epidemiological result of the rise in women smoking since the 1940s. Smoking remains the "single most important preventable cause of death" in the United States (Surgeon General's Report 1989). Despite the decline the smoking, the tobacco industry remains highly profitable (Business Week 1986), and the industry continues to spend more than $2 billion each year promoting the sale of cigarettes (Davis 1987).

IMPLICATIONS FOR THE DEVELOPING WORLD

The experience of the United States makes clear that the twentieth century trend toward proliferation of the cigarette is certainly not immutable. Nor is cigarette smoking a required mark of modernity, affluence, or of the health transition. Despite a powerful industry with significant economic clout; despite a public health service with little funds; despite the positive culture values traditionally associated with smoking; there has been a revolution in social attitudes and a remarkable decline in consumption. It is worth reiterating that this change was not merely the result of a growing perception of the risks of smoking and a recognition of susceptibility to disease. Although this certainly was important, it would be difficult to overestimate the significance of a dramatic shift in the social meaning of the cigarette and the general cultural environment in which Americans smoke.

As this chapter has shown, the decline in cigarette smoking in the United States has been the result of a complex combination of particular scientific, social, and political forces. These forces led, over time, not only to a fundamental shift in the ways in which the risks of smoking were perceived, but—perhaps more significant—to a social environment that discredited cigarette smoking. Of what relevance is this experience for the less developed world?

A full analysis of the implications of the American experience for the developing world is obviously beyond the scope of this discussion. Nevertheless, this narrative does raise an important set of questions for considering future policy options in the developing world, where consumption has dramatically expanded in the last decades. Recent worldwide surveys of cigarette consumption show steep increases in Africa and Asia. According to the World Health Organization (WHO), there has been a 77 percent increase in consumption on the African continent in the last 25 years. In Asia and Latin America, consumption outspaced population growth by 30 percent from 1970 to 1985 (WHO 1987). The WHO recently characterized the commercial market of cigarettes in developing nations as "intense and ruthless" (Herman 1989). Moreover, cigarettes produced and marketed for the less developed countries tend to have significantly higher yields of tar, nicotine, and carbon monoxide than cigarettes marketed in the United States or Europe (Roemer 1983). According to WHO, 600,000 new cases of lung cancer now occur world-wide very year; most are the result of cigarette smoking. By the year 2000, the annual number of lung cancer cases may be as high as 2 million, with 900,000 in China alone (Chandler 1986). Nevertheless, many nations have apparently opted for the short run revenues derived from the sales of tobacco; in Brazil, for example, 12 percent of annual tax revenues are derived from tobacco. Tobacco is grown and processed in over 100 developing countries (Fielding 1985).

Given that the United States has, in fact, had considerable success in controlling cigarette smoking, it is a bitter irony that this decline has been accompanied by a rise in the volume of U.S. export sales of tobacco throughout the developing world. In this sense, the problem of tobacco consumption truly is global; changes in western consumption have been a catalyst for accelerating sales in the developing world (Schmeisser 1988).

The burden of disease inflicted by cigarette smoking need not, however, be an aspect of the health transition. Developing the political "will" to address the risks of cigarette smoking is obviously a complex and contested process (Richmond and Kotelchuck 1985). While each nation will need to develop politically viable and culturally appropriate approaches to limit consumption, the American experience may point to a set of significant variables. The authority of the vast epidemiological evidence of the hazards of smoking can be enlisted in the development of institutional mechanisms to regulate health risks. Efforts to raise the price of cigarettes as well as to create disincentives to growing tobacco require additional exploration. Greater recognition that the political and economic conflicts surrounding tobacco may be powerfully influenced by the cultural meaning of the cigarette may serve to generate new strategies in utilizing the media for health promotion. Because of the multinational nature of the tobacco industry, trade and diplomatic efforts to restrict sales must be developed. Public health agencies will need to directly challenge the positive meanings of the cigarette promulgated by these corporations. Nations producing cigarettes must weigh the short-term economic gains against the serious impact on morbidity and mortality.

As the history of the health transition in the United States makes clear, patterns of health are influenced by a range of variables: biological, social, economic, and political. While this is obviously a truism, it nevertheless reflects a reality concerning the nature of the forces that influence the risks of disease and the possibilities of health. A clear recognition of these forces—and the nature of their interaction—offers real hope for reducing the burden of disease.

NOTE

This project was supported in part by BRSG–2-S07 RR 05381–27 awarded by the Biomedical Research Support Grant Program, Division of Research Resources, National Institutes of Health. Portions of this chapter initially appeared in and were adapted by permission of *Daedalus*, Journal of the American Academy of Arts and Sciences, from "The Cigarette, Risk, and American Culture," *Risk*, 119:1 (Fall 1990): 155–76.

REFERENCES

Bennett, W. 1980. The Cigarette Century. *Science* 80:37–43.

Burney, L. E. 1959. Smoking and Lung Cancer: A Statement of the Public Health Service. *Journal of the American Medical Association* 71:1829–37.

Business Week. 1986. Tobacco Company Profits Just Won't Quit. December 22:66–67.

———. 1987. No Smoking Sweeps America. July 27:40–47.

Chandler, W. U. 1986. *Banishing Tobacco*. World Watch Paper 68. Washington, D.C.: World Watch Institute.

Cornfield, J. 1959. Smoking and Lung Cancer: Recent Evidence and Discussion of Some Questions. *Journal of the National Cancer Institute* 22:123–203.

Davis, R. M. 1987. Current Trends in Cigarette Advertising and Marketing. *New England Journal of Medicine* 316:12:725–32.

Doll, R., and A. B. Hill. 1952. A Study of the Aetiology of Carcinoma of the Lung. *British Medical Journal* 2:1271–86.

———. 1954. The Mortality of Doctors in Relation to Their Smoking Habits: A Preliminary Report. *British Medical Journal* 1:4877:1451–55.

———. 1956. Lung Cancer and Other Causes of Death in Relation to Smoking: A Second Report on the Mortality of British Doctors. *British Medical Journal* 2:1071–81.

Feinstein, A. R. 1967. *Clinical Judgment*. Baltimore: Williams and Wilkins.

Fielding, J. E. 1985. Smoking: Health Effects and Control. *New England Journal of Medicine* 313:8:491–98; 313:9:555–61.

Fielding, J. E., and F. J. Phenow. 1988. Health Effects of Involuntary Smoking. *New England Journal of Medicine* 319:22:1452–60.

Fiore, M. C., T. E. Novotny, J. P. Pierce, K. M. Hatziandreu, and R. M. Davis. Trends in Cigarette Smoking in the United States: The Changing Influence of Gender and Race. *Journal of the American Medical Association* 261:49–55.

Fisher, R. A. 1957. Alleged Dangers of Cigarette-Smoking. *British Medical Journal* 2:43:297–98.

Fox, R. W., and T. J. Lears. 1983. *The Culture of Consumption*. New York: Pantheon.

Fritschler, A. L. 1969. *Smoking and Politics: Policymaking and the Federal Bureaucracy*. New York: Appleton-Century-Crofts.

Hammond, C. 1962. The Effects of Smoking. *Scientific American* 20:39–51.

Hammond, E. C., and D. Horn. 1958a. Smoking and Death Rates—Report on

Forty-four Months of Follow-Up in 187,783 Men. I: Total Mortality. *Journal of the American Medical Association* 166:10:1159–72.

―――. 1958b. Smoking and Death Rates—Report on Forty-four Months of Follow-Up on 187,783 Men. II: Death Rates by Cause. *Journal of the American Medical Association* 166:11:1294–1308.

Henningfield, J. E. 1984. Pharmacologic Basis and Treatment of Cigarette Smoking. *Clinical Psychiatry* 45:24–34.

Herman, R. 1989. Diseases of Affluence. *Washington Post Health* (January 3):12–15.

Hoffman, F. L. 1931. Cancer and Smoking Habits. *Annals of Surgery* (January):50–67.

Iglehart, J. K. 1984. Smoking and Public Policy. *New England Journal of Medicine* 310:8:539–44.

―――. 1986. The Campaign against Smoking Gains Momentum. *New England Journal of Medicine* 314:16:1059–64.

Knowles, J. 1977. The Responsibility of the Individual. *Daedalus* 106:57–80.

Leventhal, H., and P. D. Cleary. 1980. The Smoking Problem: A Review of the Research and Theory in Behavioral Risk Modification. *Psychological Bulletin* 88:2:370–405.

Lilienfeld, A. M. 1983. The Surgeon General's "Epidemiological Criteria for Causality." *Journal of Chronic Diseases* 36:837–45.

Little, C. C. 1961. Some Phases of the Problem of Smoking and Lung Cancer. *New England Journal of Medicine* 264:1241–45.

Lombard, H. L., and C. R. Doering. 1928. Cancer Studies in Massachusetts, 2: Habits, Characteristics, and Environment of Individuals with and without Cancer. *New England Journal of Medicine* 198:481–87.

MacKay, J. 1989. Battlefield for the Tobacco War. *Journal of the American Medical Association* 261:28–29.

Marchand, R. 1985. *Advertising the American Dream.* Berkeley: University of California Press.

Muller, M. 1983. Preventing Tomorrow's Epidemic: The Control of Smoking and Tobacco Production in Developing Countries. *New York State Journal of Medicine* 83:1304–1309.

Ochsner, A. 1973. My First Recognition of the Relationship of Smoking and Lung Cancer. *Preventive Medicine* 2:611–14.

Pearl, R. 1938. Tobacco Smoking and Longevity. *Science* 87:2252:216–17.

Pertschuk, M. 1982. *Revolt against Regulation: The Rise and Pause of the Consumer Movement.* Berkeley: University of California Press.

―――. 1986. *The Giant Killers.* New York: W. W. Norton.

Pierce, J. P., M. C. Fiore, T. E. Novotny, E. J. Hatziandreu, and R. M. Davis. Trends in Cigarette Smoking in the United States: Education Differences Are Increasing. *Journal of the American Medical Association* 261:56–60.

Ravenholt, R. T. 1985. Tobacco's Impact on Twentieth-Century U.S. Mortality Patterns. *American Journal of Preventive Medicine* 1:4–17.

Richmond, J. B., and M. Kotelchuck. 1985. Co-Ordination and Development of Strategies and Policy for Public Health Promotion in the United States. In *Textbook of Public Health*, vol. 2. W. W. Holland, R. Detels, and E. G. Knox, eds. London: Oxford Press.

Roemer, R. 1983. *Legislative Action to Combat the World Smoking Epidemic.* Geneva: World Health Organization.

Sapolsky, H. M. 1980. The Political Obstacles to the Control of Cigarettes in the United States. *Journal of Health Politics, Policy and Law* 5:2:277–90.

Schmeisser, P. 1988. Pushing Cigarettes Overseas. *New York Times Magazine* (July 10):16–25.

Schudson, M. 1985. *Advertising, the Uneasy Persuasion.* New York: Basic Books.

Sobel, R. 1978. *They Satisfy: The Cigarette in American Life.* New York: Doubleday.

Surgeon General's Advisory Committee Papers. 1964. National Archives Manuscripts. Washington, D.C.

Surgeon General's Report. 1964. *Smoking and Health Report of the Advisory Committee to the Surgeon General of the Public Health Service.* PHS Publication No. 1103. Washington, D.C.: U.S. Department of Health, Education, and Welfare, Public Health Service.

———. 1980. *The Health Consequences of Smoking for Women.* DHHS Publication No. D–326–003. Washington, D.C.: U.S. Department of Health and Human Services. Public Health Service.

———. 1986. *The Health Consequences of Involuntary Smoking.* DHHS Publication No. (CDC) 87–8398. Washington, D.C.: U.S. Department of Health and Human Services, Public Health Service.

———. 1988. *The Health Consequences of Smoking: Nicotine Addiction.* DHHS Publication No. (CDC) 88–8406. Washington, D.C.: U.S. Department of Health and Human Services, Public Health Service.

———. 1989. *Reducing the Health Consequences of Smoking. Twenty-Five Years of Progress.* DHHS Publication No. (CDC) 90–8411. Washington, D.C.: U.S. Department of Health and Human Services, Public Health Service.

Terry, L. 1983. The First Surgeon General's Report on Smoking. *New York State Journal of Medicine* 83:13:1254–55.

Troyer, R. J., and G. E. Marle. 1983. *The Battle over Smoking.* New Brunswick, N.J.: Rutgers University Press.

Wagner, S. 1971. *Cigarette Country.* New York: Praeger Publishers.

Wall Street Journal. 1988. Surgeon General's Stature Is Likely to Add Force to Report on Smoking as Addiction. (May 13)2:1.

Warner, K. E. 1977. The Effects of the Anti-Smoking Campaign on Cigarette Consumption. *American Journal of Public Health* 67:645–50.

———. 1981. Cigarette Smoking the 1970s: The Impact of the Anti-Smoking Campaign on Consumption. *Science* 211:729–31.

———. 1985. Cigarette Advertising and Media Coverage of Smoking and Health. *New England Journal of Medicine* 312:384–88.

Washington Post. 1989. U.S. Report Raises Estimate of Smoking Toll. January 11:A20.

Whelan, E., M. 1984. *A Smoking Gun.* Philadelphia: George F. Stickley Co.

Whiteside, T. 1971. *Selling Death: Cigarette Advertising and Public Health.* New York: Liveright.

World Health Organization. 1983. *Smoking Control Strategies in Developing Countries.* Technical Report, Series 695. Geneva and Washington, D.C.: WHO.

————. 1987. *Tobacco Alert*. 20 (April–June):3.

Wynder, E. L., and E. A. Graham. 1950. Tobacco Smoking as a Possible Etiologic Factor in Bronchiogenic Carcinoma: A Study of 684 Proved Cases. *Journal of the American Medical Association* 143:329–96.

Commentary: Tobacco Use in India

PRAKASH C. GUPTA

Tobacco use has been widely recognized as the major preventable cause of death and disease in the world today. While the use of tobacco in cigars, pipes, and also in smokeless form is not uncommon in the industrialized world, the predominance of cigarette smoking means that discussions of health or economic issues related to tobacco consumption tend to focus exclusively on cigarettes. Brandt's Chapter, "The Rise and Fall of the Cigarette: A Brief History of the Antismoking Movement in the United States," is an illustration of this.

In India, however, cigarettes represent only a minor fraction of overall tobacco use. India has the second largest population in the world and has been a major producer and consumer of tobacco for several decades. Thus, special attention needs to be given to India in any global assessment of the health problems of tobacco use.

In discussing the possible health consequences of tobacco in India, we have to consider the wide spectrum of tobacco use that prevails there (Mehta, Pindborg, Gupta, and Daftary, 1969). The most common and widespread form of tobacco smoking in India is not cigarettes but *bidi*. Bidi is handmade in the following way. First, 0.15 to 0.25 gm of coarsely ground tobacco is placed on a dried rectangular piece of *temburni* lead (diospyros melanoxylon). This is then rolled into a slight conical shape and secured with thread. The length of bidi varies from 4 cm to 8 cm.

Although bidi contains much less tobacco than cigarettes, it is at least, if not more, damaging in terms of tar and nicotine delivery. Bidi is also much cheaper than cigarettes. A bidi costs less than one-tenth of a cigarette, which means that bidi are smoked by the poorer sections of society. Bidi are advertised, but not in a high profile, glossy manner as cigarettes are.

The bidi industry has considerable economic and political clout because it generates employment, especially for the rural poor. The temburni leaves for bidi are collected from the forest by tribal people. Handrolling of bidi is done by rural poor, especially women. Thus, bidi generates employment for several million individuals in the economically weaker sections of Indian society.

Bidi is smoked mostly by men. It is popular in all parts of India. Cigarettes are smoked mostly by members of the urban middle class, who are comparatively affluent. Other forms of tobacco use are popular in specific areas. *Chutta*, for example, is a handmade cheroot that is popular in the southeastern parts of India. In certain coastal areas it may be smoked in a reverse manner, that is, by keeping the glowing end inside the mouth. Women are especially likely to smoke chutta in this way. In Srikakulam district on the east coast, for example, 60 percent of women aged 15 years or older were reported to be reverse chutta smokers (Pindborg, Mehta, Gupta, Daftary, and Smith, 1971).

Tobacco was brought to India in the sixteenth century and smoked in hubble-bubble (water pipes) in Mogul courts. Tobacco smoking in hubble-bubble is still a common practice in several parts of northern India among both men and women. Clay pipes are smoked in the western region of India, while in Goa *dhumti* smoking is practiced. Dhumti is a form of bidi that uses different kinds of leaves for wrapping tobacco (Bhonsle, Murti, Gupta, and Mehta 1976).

Smokeless tobacco use in India is more varied. The most common habit is betel quid chewing. Betel quid chewing dates back at least 2,000 years in India. It is a part of religious and cultural rituals and enjoys complete social acceptance.

Traditionally, betel quid consisted of betel leaf, pieces of areca nut, a few drops of lime (calcium hydroxide), several condiments, and sweetening and flavoring agents that reflected regional practices and individual preferences. Although tobacco was introduced in India primarily as a substance for smoking, it also became an ingredient of betel quid. By becoming associated with a socially accepted practice, smokeless tobacco use became widespread. Now, almost all habitual consumers of betel quid use it with tobacco. This habit is widespread in all parts of India and is practiced by both men and women.

The next most popular practice involves *khaini*, which is a mixture of tobacco and lime. Consumption of khaini is common in many parts of India but may be known by different names in different areas. *Mawa* is a combination of tobacco, lime, and areca nut that is popular in western regions. Oral use of manufactured snuff is also common in the western regions. *Mishri* is a powdered form of roasted tobacco that is common in Maharashtra and the central regions of India, especially among women.

Tobacco is also mixed with molasses and used in the form of paste. The paste is known as *gudakhu*. Gudakhu use is common in the eastern region. Creamy snuff is a manufactured item marketed in toothpaste-like tubes. It is reported to be common in Goa.

The most recent arrival upon the smokeless tobacco scene is *pan masala*. Pan masala is a manufactured item containing areca nut and other ingredients common in betel quid. It is available in two forms: with or without tobacco. Since there are no restrictions on advertising a nontobacco product, pan masala without tobacco is vigorously promoted, even on electronic media. Since pan masala with tobacco carries the same brand name, it benefits equally from this unrestricted advertising.

The health consequences of all these tobacco products have been investigated only to a limited extent (Sanghvi and Notani 1989). One of the most common cancers in India is oral cancer. Many of the forms of tobacco use described here, especially the smokeless ones, have been investigated for association with oral cancer and precancerous lesions. All show a very strong association. When standard epidemiologic criteria are applied to the available data, the relationship can be concluded to be causal (International Agency for Research on Cancer 1984).

Smokeless tobacco use has also been associated with cancer of other parts of the upper aerodigestive tract. It has not been investigated for possible association with other diseases.

. Bidi smoking has been shown to be associated with cancers of the oral cavity, lungs, pharynx, larynx, and esophagus. It also increases the risk of heart disease and decreases lung function. Chutta smoking is strongly associated with cancer of the oral cavity, especially of the palate; it has also been shown to decrease lung function.

The health consequences of tobacco use in India have been assessed by looking at the overall relative risk of mortality among tobacco users in a cohort study of two regions. In one area, where bidi smoking and betel quid chewing were prevalent, the age-adjusted excess risk was significantly (30 percent) higher among smokes. It is surprising that even among chewers the excess risk was 20. This too was significant; however, lack of information precluded any conclusions about the specific causes of this excess mortality except in the case of oral cancer (Gupta, Bhonsle, Mehta, and Pindborg 1984). In another areas, where reverse smoking was practiced, the age-adjusted excess mortality was close to 100 percent (Gupta, Mehta, and Pindborg, 1984).

An attempt has been made to assess the overall health consequences of tobacco consumption by estimating the morality attributable to tobacco use. It has been estimated that every year 630,000 adult deaths are attributable to tobacco usage in India (Gupta 1988). Due to lack of information, it is possible to categorize only 56 percent of these excess deaths according to cause of death (Notani, Jayant, and Sanghvi 1989).

Can these tobacco habits in rural populations be changed by educational efforts, and would such efforts result in health benefits? An answer to this question has been provided by an intervention study among rural Indian populations in three areas of India. Over 36,000 tobacco users were interviewed for tobacco use and examined for the presence of oral cancer and precancerous lesions. All these individuals were given health education regarding the ill effects of tobacco use through both personal communication and the use of the mass media. Personal communication was provided by the examining dentist and a social scientist. Use of the mass media included documentary films, posters, newspaper articles, radio messages, and folk-art theater.

Considerable social science research was carried out to investigate the reasons why people began using tobacco, why they continued to use it, what they perceived as the effects of using tobacco, and what input might help them to discontinue this behavior. The results of the research were fed back into the educational process.

The educational campaign and accompanying interviews and examinations were carried out once a year. An assessment after five years of follow-up showed that significantly higher percentages of individuals in the intervention cohort stopped or reduced their tobacco use compared to controls. As a consequence, the incidence of precancerous lesions decreased substantially in the intervention cohort (Gupta, Mehta, Pindborg, Aghi, Bhonsle, Murti, Daftary, Shah, and Sinor 1986). Similar results were reported after eight years of follow-up (Gupta, Mehta, Pindborg, Daftary, Aghi, Bhonsle, and Murti 1990).

This discussion is intended to point out that the problem of tobacco use in India is quite different from the situation in industrialized countries. The health consequences of tobacco use in India are very serious but not as well understood as in the industrialized world. We do know, however, that it is possible to educate the population regarding the ill effects of tobacco use, and that such an effort would result in a health benefit to the population.

It is well recognized that a major transition in the health status of human populations would result from a change in tobacco use behavior. Brandt's chapter documents the nature and process of this change in the United States. In India, the feasibility of initiating such a change has been demonstrated. It is clear that in initiating as well as in accelerating these changes, social science research and applications will continue to play a major role.

REFERENCES

Bhonsle, R. B., P. R. Murti, P. C. Gupta, and F. S. Mehta. 1976. Reverse Dhumti Smoking in Goa: An Epidemiologic Study of 5,449 Villagers for Oral Precancerous Lesions. *Indian Journal of Cancer* 13:301–5.

Gupta, P. C. 1988. Health Consequences of Tobacco Use in India. *World Smoking and Health* 13:5–10.

Gupta, P. C., R. B. Bhonsle, F. S. Mehta, and J. J. Pindborg. 1984. Mortality Experience in Relation to Tobacco Chewing and Smoking Habits from a Ten-Year Follow-Up Study in Ernakulam District, Kerala. *International Journal of Epidemiology* 13:184–87.

Gupta, P. C., F. S. Mehta, and J. J. Pindborg. 1984. Mortality among Reverse Chutta Smokers in South India. *British Medical Journal* 289:865–66.

Gupta, P. C., F. S. Mehta, J. J. Pindborg, M. B. Aghi, R. B. Bhonsle, P. R. Murti, D. K. Daftary, H. T. Shah, and P. N. Sinor. 1986. Intervention Study for Primary Prevention of Oral Cancer among 36,000 Indian Tobacco Users. *Lancet* 1:1235–38.

Gupta, P. C., F. S. Mehta, J. J. Pindborg, D. K. Daftary, M. B. Aghi, R. B. Bhonsle, and P. R. Murti, 1990. A Primary Prevention Study of Oral Cancer among Indian Villagers: Eight-Year-Follow-Up Results. In *Evaluating Effectiveness of Primary Prevention of Cancer*. M. Hakama, V. Beral, J. W. Culln, and D. M. Parkin, eds. IARC Scientific Publication Series No. 103. Lyon: International Agency for Research on Cancer.

International Agency for Research on Cancer. 1984. *Tobacco Habits Other than Smoking; Betel-Quid and Areca-Nut Chewing; and Some Related Nitrosamines*. IRAC Monographs on the Evaluation of the Carcinogenic Risk of Chemicals to Humans, Vol. 37. Lyon: International Agency for Research on Cancer.

Mehta, F. S., J. J. Pindborg, P. C. Gupta, and D. K. Daftary. 1969. Epidemiologic and Histologic Study of Oral Cancer and Leukoplakia among 50,915 Villagers in India. *Cancer* 24:832–49.

Notani, P. N., K. Jayant, and L. D. Sanghvi. 1989. Assessment of Morbidity and Mortality Due to Tobacco Usage in India. In *Tobacco and Health—The Indian Scene, 1989*. L. D. Sanghvi and P. Notani, eds. Bombay: International Union against Cancer—Tata Memorial Centre.

Pindborg, J. J., F. S. Mehta, P. C. Gupta, D. K. Daftary, and C. J. Smith. 1971. Reverse Smoking in Andhra Pradesh, India: A Study of Palatal Lesions among 10,169 Villagers. *British Journal of Cancer* 25:10–20.

Sanghvi, L. D., and P. Notani, eds. 1989. *Tobacco and Health—The Indian Scene, 1989*. Bombay: International Union against Cancer—Tata Memorial Centre.

5

Using Social Science to Prevent and Control HIV Infection: The Experience of Britain, Sweden, and the United States

DANIEL M. FOX

Social scientists often complain that many of the people who make and implement health policy ignore or resist the results of their research. The short history of the epidemic of HIV infection provides evidence that policymakers, particularly elected officials and the people they appoint, also have a reasonable complaint: Why do so many social scientists ignore or resist the difficulties of making and implementing policy?

Both complaints miss the fundamental point, which is that social scientists and policymakers interested in preventing or controlling AIDS or any other disease confront the same problem: how to achieve particular goals in a particular environment. For people who live their professional lives in either politics or applied social science, these goals include surviving, prospering, and making a difference. The environments in which they try to achieve these goals are shaped by the values, beliefs, and institutions of national, regional, local cultures.

Each country has the health policy it deserves. Put more politely, each country's health policy is a result of the ways in which ideas about illness and how to address it—ideas that have often transcended national boundaries in this century—have been refracted by its political culture (Fox 1986). This is not determinism. Rather, I am urging social scientists to take more seriously the negotiations about the causes, diagnosis, prevention, and treatment of disease that take place within particular countries and, and particular, in their political systems or cultures.

The first questions to ask about a policy in a particular country are (1) how and by whom it was initiated, and (2) why it does what—to, for, and with, whom. Unfortunately, many social scientists concerned about health policy have preferred to ask different questions, because they assume that expertise, or sometimes ideology, has granted us special knowledge about what policy in a particular country ought to be. For example, there is a large body of literature inquiring about why the United States lacks comprehensive national health insurance, or why the United Kingdom does not spend more of its national product on medical care, or why Sweden has a relatively weak private medical care sector. Similar normative assumptions have also influenced discussions about policy during the HIV epidemic—stimulating, for instance, queries about why the United State has not embraced needle exchanges, or Britain not been eager to conduct blinded seroprevalence surveys, or Sweden not been sympathetic to methadone maintenance for its heroin addicts. Such questions can, at times, help to clarify national differences and similarities. But they are subordinate to the problems of understanding the history and present situation of policy in particular countries.

Drawing upon my experience with interventions to prevent and control HIV infection in the United States and, to a lesser extent, in Sweden and the United Kingdom, I address here three distinct questions. All are central to understanding both policy and the role of social science in influencing and understanding it. These questions are:

- How important is the prevention and control of HIV infection in the policy and politics of each country?
- What do policymakers in each country believe they know about preventing and controlling diseases?
- Who usually does what to, for, and with whom to prevent and control diseases in each country, and is HIV infection a special case?

THE IMPORTANCE OF HIV INFECTION

The importance of a disease in the health policy of any country is only in part a result of its rates of incidence, prevalence, and case-fatality. By the end of 1988, the cumulative incidence of AIDS in the United States (237.7 cases per million population) was an order of magnitude greater than in Britain (which had an incidence of 25.2 million) and Sweden (21.5 million). Yet the epidemic is regarded as a major problem of health policy, requiring extraordinary measures, in all three countries. In all three, moreover, the policies and politics of AIDS attract considerable attention from the media. In all three there there was initial surprise, that, contrary to the expectations of officials, the medical community, and the general public, an infectious disease was not easily controllable by the methods of biological, clinical, and social science. Within the previous generation, chronic disease had become the preoccupation of health policy in all three countries. Similarly, in all three there was concern about the potential spread of HIV infection from homosexual men and intravenous drug users to what many people are pleased to call the "general population" (Fox, Day, and Klein 1989).

These similarities are reflected in the policies of the three countries. In all three, initial government reaction to AIDS was slow and cautious, even dilatory to some critics. When the central governments in Britain and Sweden decided to take strong initiatives in 1985–1986, they quickly and effectively dominated debate and established consensus about the importance of the epidemic. Although events in the United States have been considerably more contentious, federal and state policy have accorded high priority to AIDS, especially since 1985.

Nevertheless, there are important differences in how the epidemic has been perceived in each country. The importance or relative priority of the epidemic in each country's policy is a result of who is perceived to be at risk of what, and of who presses particular perceptions with the greatest success.

In Britain, although the disease has been mainly a phenomenon of two metropolitan areas, London and Edinburgh, the perception of risk has shifted. Public officials and the media initially presented HIV disease as a problem of deviant minorities. Since 1986 they have presented it as a threat to the general population, an opportunity to educate the public about sexual activity and drug use, and a way to increase appropriations for medical research and the National Health Service. This change occurred not as a result of a sudden surge in cases of disease, or in response to the cumulative burden of managing and paying for care, but rather in response to factors in the political environment. These factors included: (1) press coverage of "lurid AIDS stories," particularly in the tabloids, (2) the combined pressure on the government from civil servants in the health department and from external groups (especially medical and scientific interests, but also gay rights activists), and (3) a trip to the United States from which the secretary of state for health returned "very chastened" (Day and Klein 1989). British policymakers now regard HIV and its consequences as a major problem, one that is not usually compared with other diseases in incidence, potential threat, or cost.

The importance of the epidemic has been much more controversial in Sweden, both before and since the central government's policy initiatives of 1985. Before 1985, many prominent gays as well as leaders of academic medicine worried in public about exaggerating the importance of the disease. The gays were concerned about discrimination; the academics about the deflection of resources from research and patient care for what they regarded as more important diseases. More recently, other critics have worried that HIV infection is a distraction from the priorities of

Swedish drug abuse policies. In addition, there has been concern about oversaturating the public with warnings. Some academics still complain about the deflection of resources (Fox, Day, and Klein 1989).

The fragmentation of health policy in the United States makes it more difficult to characterize the importance accorded to the epidemic in health policy. For example, the federal government has made HIV a priority for research and is spending more money on it than for any disease except cancer. But it has spent relatively modestly for prevention and has, in general, left the problems of organizing and financing treatment to states, municipalities, and the private sector (Fox 1989a). The states with the largest number of cases—New York, California, New Jersey, and Florida—have accorded the most importance to the epidemic. By 1988, however, cases had been reported from every state. Rates of incidence were increasing the fastest in states with the largest black and Hispanic populations. Legislators and executive branch officials in the states were now defining the epidemic as mainly a phenomenon of minority groups and were, for the first time in several years, wondering in public about how to balance financing for the control of HIV with their other responsibilities (Fox 1988a).

In all three countries, the importance accorded the epidemic has been more a result of perceived threat than of the number of cases of disease. Even in the United States, especially outside New York City and San Francisco, many other diseases place greater pressures on the resources available for prevention and treatment.

Moreover, the importance accorded to the epidemic, and how relative priority has been expressed in policy, must be interpreted in the context of the political institutions of each country. In Britain, HIV infection has been accommodated within established policies that have broad public support and are nonpartisan. The acrimony about the importance of the epidemic between 1982 and 1985 threatened the standard processes of achieving consensus on health and social policy in Sweden. Swedish officials established an extraordinary national commission to restore that consensus (Fox, Day, and Klein 1989). In the United States, the importance accorded HIV infection has been influenced by two issues—race and health care financing—that are not central to policy for the epidemic in Europe. Moreover, the epidemic in the United States coincided with what I have called a "crisis of authority" in health affairs in the United States. The elements in this crisis included pressures to shift the locus of authority for health policy from the federal government to the states and the private sector, decreasing willingness of public officials to let physicians and scientists continue to control spending with minimal oversight, and the strength of right-wing pressure groups whose views precluded sympathy for a disease that was most prevalent among hom-

osexual men and intravenous drug users and that afflicted a dispropor-
tionate number of blacks and Hispanics (Fox 1988b).

In all three countries, for different reasons, there has been resistance
to proposed policies and research activities that would establish more
precisely the present and potential importance of the epidemic. In Britain, for example, where there is a long tradition of according absolute
priority to the confidentiality of the doctor-patient relationship, and thus
of voluntary reporting of venereal disease on a confidential basis, there
has been considerable opposition to mandatory reporting of infection
(Porter and Porter 1988). Only at the end of 1988 did anonymous testing
of routine blood samples begin in Britain. In Sweden, there is vigorous
opposition among physicians, and apparently much noncompliance,
with a 1985 law requiring that positive tests for HIV infection be noted
in medical records and that doctors initiate contact-tracing. Physicians
who do not want to risk stigmatizing their patients often omit pertinent
information from medical records, particularly when the patients with
HIV infection are health care providers. In the United States, there has
been considerable acrimony about the propriety and likelihood of success
of research to learn more about the prevalence of infection and of sexual
behavior that would encourage its spread. There is also growing support
in the United States for mandatory (the euphemism is "routine") testing
for HIV in newborns, for candidates for surgery, and for health professionals who perform invasive procedures.

The problems of devising, implementing, and evaluating policy about
the epidemic have not been subject to much research in either national
or comparative studies. Only a few social scientists in the three countries
are trying to understand systematically the policies that respond to the
epidemic. Explaining this situation is beyond the scope of this chapter.
Part of the explanation, however, involves the issue addressed in the
next section: what people in the health professions, and in particular
public health, believe they know about preventing and controlling infectious disease.

PREVENTING AND CONTROLLING INFECTIOUS DISEASE

When AIDS was first recognized in 1981, public health officials in the
United States and western Europe were confident that most of the problems of controlling infectious disease had been solved. Four major components of infectious disease control were in place: surveillance,
research, prevention, and treatment. Each of these methods had been
brought to a considerable level of sophistication and apparent effectiveness during the twentieth century. Infectious diseases had ceased to be

the major causes of death almost half a century earlier. Epidemiology, laboratory science, and clinical medicine had combined with rising standards of living to shift the priorities of public health from infection to chronic disease. In the United States, the Centers for Disease Control had just a few years earlier provided an excellent case study in effective infectious disease control in the work that resolved the problems of what was called Legionnaire's Disease (Fox 1988a).

Although this was the dominant view among people responsible for public health policy, there were undercurrents of doubt. Scientific understanding of viral infections was increasing rapidly, but so were surprising discoveries (Grmek 1989). Some of the limits of surveillance and vaccine technology became apparent to a broad public in the events surrounding the nonepidemic of swine influenza in 1976 (Silverstein 1981). Since the 1950s, a growing number of researchers, using data from historical epidemiology, had questioned the assumption that scientific advances and public health practice were responsible for declining mortality from infectious disease since the nineteenth century.

Recent experience in controlling chronic disease had, however, strengthened the confidence of the people who made and implemented public health policy. The declining incidence of cardiovascular disease appeared to be attributable to changes in eating and exercise habits resulting from educational campaigns. In the United States, especially, programs to persuade people to stop smoking cigarettes were associated with declining incidence of diseases of the heart and lungs.

The historical analogies that experts in public health, in both government and universities, have used to describe the HIV epidemic to each other and the public reveal a great deal about their attitude toward policy. For most of the 1980s, in all three countries they most often compared AIDS to bubonic plague, cholera, and yellow fever. Epidemics of these diseases had sudden and rapid onset, afflicted people of all social classes, had high rates of mortality, and subsided after a few months or years. Policy for reacting to them before the twentieth century included declaring states of emergency, mobilizing lay and medical authority outside the normal channels of government, isolating and quarantining victims and suspected carriers, and making extraordinary public expenditures. In the twentieth century the incidence of these diseases had declined, most officials and historians agreed, because science, surveillance, prevention, and treatment had reduced them to almost negligible threats (Fee and Fox 1989).

These analogies were more comforting than others that were mentioned, but with less frequency, to tuberculosis, venereal disease, and leprosy. These infectious diseases were endemic and required facilities and expenditures for long-term as well as acute care. They persisted in populations for centuries. Researchers had identified the microorganisms that carry these diseases and had devised treatments for them, but prevention and treatment were compromised by behavioral, social, and economic factors, including the stigmatization of those afflicted with them (Brandt 1987).

Neither the medical nor the social sciences offered ready answers to the major questions of public policy for preventing and controlling the HIV epidemic. Officials reposed confidence in the methods of public health mainly because of the association between policies and the declining incidence of infectious disease for over more than a century. In particular, research on surveillance—including both reporting and testing—and on prevention—by individual counseling and mass education—offered very little guidance for public policy. There was considerable evidence of erratic reporting of diseases that carried stigma and of the ineffectiveness of mandatory screening in the absence of simple and effective treatments (Fox 1987). Very little could be claimed with any statistical confidence about the effects of different educational interventions on behavior.

What little was known about controlling disease as a result of social science has, in general, influenced policy in all three countries. For example, procedures have been designed to compensate for underreporting. Testing and counseling have been linked and have, in general, been voluntary. Education has been targeted to particular groups, although, for sound political reasons in each country, much of it has been aimed at general audiences.

The lack of systematic knowledge in the applied social sciences that was sufficiently persuasive to guide policies for disease control had been a problem in all three countries long before the AIDS epidemic. Laboratory and clinical research had received priority in public funding throughout the century. Few of the social and behavioral scientists who worked on problems of disease surveillance and prevention had much prestige either in the health professions or among their colleagues in academic disciplines.

The largest body of social science research on issues of importance to health policy was largely irrelevant to the initial problems of the HIV epidemic. Many studies of the costs and utilization of health services had been conducted, mainly in the United States, since the 1960s. This research had been stimulated by growing costs and uneven access to services. It had little bearing on countries where health services were a universal entitlement paid out of general tax revenues or mandatory insurance payments and where data were less readily available because they were not required to generate bills to patients or to third-party payers. Moreover, reflecting the priorities of health policy in the United States, researchers concentrated on access to treatment and the cost-effectiveness of health services rather than on prevention.

Policy for prevention and control was, therefore, usually made on the basis of expertise rather than science in all three countries. This is not an unusual situation for policy in other areas, such as defense, education, or the economy. It seemed unusual in health affairs because of the widely shared assumption in all three countries that medical science could (and with enough funding, would) answer most of the outstanding questions about diseases and their control. Partly as a result of this powerful assumption, health officials are more reluctant than their colleagues in other areas of public affairs to admit the lack of a scientific basis for their policy choices.

The absence of a scientific basis for policy to control a highly visible epidemic has exposed public health officials in all three countries to unaccustomed criticism. In all three, civil libertarians and gay rights advocates have challenged particular policies for testing and reporting. Feminist groups in Sweden have objected to the effects of testing policies on prostitutes. In all three, moreover (though mainly in the United States), public education policies have been criticized by groups opposed to explicit descriptions of gay or heterosexual sex. In Sweden and the United States there has been controversy over policies to control HIV among intravenous drug users—notably needle sharing and simplified methadone maintenance programs—that do not take account of larger issues of control and therapy (Fox, Day, and Klein 1989).

An unexpected result of almost a decade of efforts to prevent and control HIV infection in all three countries has been to remove some of the exemption from normal politics that public health has enjoyed for much of this century. This change has been most pronounced in the United States, least in Sweden. In the United States, the media now treat state and local health commissioners' pronouncements about HIV control with about the same degree of respect that is accorded to official opinions about housing, highways, and schools. Similarly, in both Britain and Sweden, elected officials and representatives of interest groups question expert opinion about disease surveillance and prevention more than they have done at any time in the century. Although health professionals still dominate policy for HIV control in all three countries, there is evidence in each that public health policy is losing its privileged political status. The next section of this chapter describes some of the consequences of the normalization of public health policy and politics.

WHO DOES WHAT TO WHOM: HIV AS NORMAL POLITICS

As we enter the second decade of the epidemic, HIV infection is having unanticipated effects on the health policies of each of the three countries. In Britain, the epidemic is testing the ability of a government that places a high value on management to respond to an administratively complicated health crisis. The ability of the National Health Service to address the highly specific needs of particular patients during a period of tension about reorganization is also being tested. In Sweden, the epidemic has revealed the boundaries of health policymaking by consensus, calling into question the continued ability of party leaders, civil servants, and representatives of interest groups to make hard choices with little public debate. In the United States, the epidemic places additional stress on health policy, especially financing policy, that is already subject to powerful and contentious advocacy for change.

The fundamental cause of these effects on health policy is that HIV has become a chronic infectious disease, one of many disabling chronic illnesses competing for resources. After almost a decade in which the number of cases has steadily increased—and the number of people infected remains unknown—it makes little sense to compare HIV disease to plague or cholera or even to influenza and infantile paralysis. The analogies to tuberculosis—the largest cause of mortality from disease in the nineteenth century—or to venereal disease grow more persuasive.

To argue that HIV has become a chronic disease is, however, not to claim that all chronic diseases are alike. HIV resembles other chronic diseases in the amount of uncertainty about how much time elapses (especially with chemotherapy) from infection to onset and from onset to death, in its claims on resources for long-term care, and in its relatively high cost per case (Fox 1989b). New treatments that increase survival time are making it even more conspicuous as a chronic problem. Yet AIDS is unlike the leading chronic diseases that are the focus of health policy in the three countries. It is not a disease of the middle and later years of life. Moreover, the sexual and needle-sharing behaviors that lead to most cases evoke less sympathy than, for example, overeating, smoking, and drinking alcoholic beverages do.

Moreover, unlike most chronic diseases, but like tuberculosis a century ago, officials in most countries can still rely on fear as a basis for policy to prevent and control HIV infection. In the late nineteenth century, policies to control tuberculosis acquired important political supporters as a result of fear among people in the middle and upper classes that the disease would be communicated to them in public places or by their servants. Fear of tuberculosis declined after 1910 as the number of new cases recorded fell each year (Fox 1975). HIV infection is likely to have a similar history. But as a result of the politics of HIV in all three countries in the 1980s, policy is less likely to be a near monopoly of the most influential health professionals than it was in the past (Fox 1990).

During the 1980s, although the dominance of professionals in health policy was reduced, they nevertheless had the most powerful influence on HIV policy in all three countries. Health professionals were more accountable to elected officials than they had been in the past. They also had to take greater account of the representatives of interest groups and were more susceptible to the agendas and the pressures of the media.

These three alternative sources of power in health affairs—elected officials, interest groups, and the media—have had different effects on HIV policy in each country. Here are a few examples, beginning with elected officials. In Britain, all-party parliamentary committees have made significant contributions to shaping and evaluating HIV policy. In Sweden, the structure of the national AIDS commission gives members of parliament from opposition parties a stronger public role in policy-making. In the United States, HIV is another of many recent examples of how the expertise and influence of congressman and their staff has increased since the mid–1970s (Fox 1990).

Interest groups are important to HIV policy, though in different ways in the three countries. In Britain and Sweden, where the central governments dominate policymaking for the epidemic, advocates for gay interests (which include both preventing discrimination and increasing resources for prevention and treatment) have substantial access to policymakers. In the United States, the influence of groups representing gays varies across states, and their impact on the national government is problematic. Moreover, leaders of black and Hispanic groups and public officials identified with them often have different priorities in drug abuse policy than officials concerned with HIV do.

The media are important in policy formation for HIV in all three countries. In each country, major newspapers and television organizations cover the science and policy issues of the epidemic in considerable detail. Other media outlets amplify any potentially sensational news about HIV infection. Innovations in science and treatment for HIV are often disseminated by the media before they have been subjected to peer review for publication in academic journals. Many AIDS conferences, including the annual international meeting, are staged as media events. In the past, media attention to medical and health issues has usually been translated by professionals into a greater claim on resources. The history of public financing for medical research in the United States is the most notable instance in point. It is not clear what the impact of media exposure will be for health policy as public confidence in the inevitable progress of medical science declines. Moreover, there is research evidence that media attention to the HIV epidemic is changing in unexpected ways. For instance, it appears to be declining in the United States but not in Britain (Gross 1989).

LESSONS FOR THE HEALTH TRANSITION

The preceding discussion of efforts to prevent and control HIV infection in three industrial countries does not offer a great deal of specific guidance for using social science research to achieve the ultimate goal of better health for all. I hope, however, that I have raised at least these propositions for consideration:

- A precondition for using social science research to achieve better health is to use it to comprehend how and why each country sets the priorities it does in health policy and between health and other areas of policy.
- The methods of social science should be used to discover what the people who make and influence health policy in each country believe to be sound knowledge, both expert wisdom and science, and how they most comfortably employ that knowledge to make policy.
- Within the boundaries of what the people who make health policy in any country consider to be pertinent science and sound politics, particular findings from the social sciences can often be incorporated in policy.
- In the HIV epidemic, the influence of legislators, interest groups, and the media on policy and public opinion and health policy has been greater than the influence of social scientists. This is not necessarily bad, since, in the absence of pertinent findings from social science research, it may be more useful to open the health policy process to new opinions and sensitivities.

What lessons can we take from alternative strategies for AIDS control in the developed countries for the developing world? The first lesson, I have insisted, is that strategies to prevent and control HIV infection cannot be abstracted from particular political cultures. What is desirable, feasible, and even scientifically valid in one culture cannot be transferred easily to another. Thus, there would be little point in advocating mandatory reporting of the names of persons with AIDS or HIV infection in Britain; yet there can be considerable voluntary reporting on an anonymous basis by doctors. Nor should anyone expect full compliance by physicians with reporting requirements in Sweden, despite what the law says. In the United States, mandatory reporting of seropositivity, which its advocates claim to be successful in Colorado and a few other states, is not—at present—politically feasible in New York or California. Similarly, evidence about the effectiveness of needle exchange programs is evaluated differently and has different political impact in particular countries. In Britain, it justifies existing policy; in Sweden, people who are central to controlling drug use see it as a distraction from more important policy concerns; and in the United States, some very influential people regard it as evidence that public health officials are naive about the causes and impact of epidemic drug abuse.

A second lesson is that the importance accorded to HIV infection, and thus to preventing and controlling it, may vary even more between developed and developing countries than it does among industrial countries. Britain and Sweden have accorded the epidemic a high priority.

It is the most visible disease in contemporary public policy in these countries, although the incidence in each is an order of magnitude less than it is in the United States (and in some developing countries). In none of the three countries has any influential official or interest group publically advocated lowering the priority on HIV in order to provide resources for another area of public policy. Some people resent the attention given to gays and drug users, but no group has acted effectively in public on the basis of this resentment, even in California where referenda made possible by the state constitution give such groups an unusual opportunity. There may be more effective political support in some developing countries for according lower priority to HIV than to other diseases or other sectors of the country.

A third potential lesson for developing countries comes not from the research that I have summarized here but rather from my experience of working on HIV-related issues with officials of state and local government in the United States, notably with legislators from various states (Fordham 1989). The precondition for being invited to work with these officials is acceptance of their rules about what is politically feasible in their environment. Along with other social scientists, I help them to discover what is known, and can be known, as a result of research using the methods of social sciences. They decide whether and how to incorporate the results of that research in their work. Which legislator or official asked what question about the scientific basis of a particular policy or expressed what informed judgment about political feasibility remains confidential.

In this work, over several years I have witnessed considerable enthusiasm among officials of state and local government about the findings of research in the social sciences as it bears on the HIV epidemic. Some of this enthusiasm has been represented in legislation enacted in, among other states, Florida and Michigan (Fox 1989b). Perhaps more important, I have documented many instances in which scientifically informed chairs of legislative health and finance committees have killed bills that would mandate the testing of particular people or the heavy-handed notification of sexual partners when there is no evidence that such measures might be effective.

What matters to these officials, I have observed, is not whether social science has "proven" that some measures to prevent, control, or organize treatment for the epidemic are better than others, but rather that they can use the results of inquiry and analysis to assist them in making political judgments. They want to know what measures have had what effects on the epidemic under what conditions and at what cost. They will then decide what measures have salience in their jurisdictions. Social science is neither better nor worse than politics to them; it is simply a different, if sometimes related, subject.

The lesson of this experience is that social science research may have the most influence on policy as a set of methods and approaches rather than as a body of knowledge. Social scientists can be involved most usefully in political processes as counselors rather than as repositories of knowledge. That may be the fate of people who deal in knowledge that is contingent on time, place, and circumstance.

Social scientists can also have another, even humbler, role in policy, whether in developed or developing countries. They are often the only people with a strong professional interest in monitoring systematically who did what to, for, and with whom—when, why, and with what effects. Information about these matters is scarce, even in the HIV epidemic, which may become the most carefully studied phenomenon in health affairs in recent times. The absence of systematic efforts to write the contemporary history of responses to the epidemic and to evaluate the results of policies in various countries contributes to my finding that little has been learned about prevention and control that can even be considered for transfer from one political culture to another. As we discuss how to use social science research to improve and accelerate the health transition in less developed countries, we should acknowledge some of the ways we have failed to use it in the United States and western Europe.

REFERENCES

Brandt, A. M. 1987. *No Magic Bullet: A Social History of Venereal Disease in the United States since 1880.* Rev. ed. New York: Oxford University Press.

Day, P., and R. Klein. 1989. *Two-Way Signals: The Case of AIDS Policy Making in Britain.* Unpublished paper prepared for the WZB Symposium, Signals for Steering Government, Berlin.

Fee, E., and D. M. Fox. 1989. The Contemporary Historiography of AIDS. *Journal of Social History* 23:2:303–14. Revised version in *AIDS: The Making of a Chronic Disease.* E. Fee and D. Fox, eds. Berkeley: University of California Press (1991).

Fordham, R. A. 1989. *The User-Liaison Program of the National Center for Health Services Research and Health Care Technology Assessment.* Unpublished paper presented at the Centre for Health Economics and Policy Analysis Conference, McMaster University, Ontario, June 1989.

Fox, D. M. 1975. Social Policy and City Politics: Compulsory Notification for Tuberculosis in New York. *Bulletin of the History of Medicine* 49:2:169–95.

———. 1986. *Health Policies, Health Politics: The Experience of Britain and America, 1911–1965.* Princeton: Princeton University Press.

———. 1987. Conflicts of Power and Values: Reporting Diseases from TB to AIDS. *Hastings Center Report* 16:6:11–16.

———. 1988a. AIDS and the American Health Polity: The History and Prospects of a Crisis of Authority. In *AIDS: The Burden of History.* Elizabeth Fee and Daniel M. Fox, eds. Berkeley: University of California Press.

————. 1988b. The New Discontinuity in American Health Policy. In *America in Theory*. D. Donaghue, ed. New York: Oxford University Press.

————. 1989a. Financing Health for Persons with HIV Infection: Guidelines for State Action. *American Journal of Law and Medicine* 16:102:223–47.

————. 1989b. Politics and Epidemiology: Financing Health Services for the Chronically Ill and Disabled, 1930–1990. *The Milbank Quarterly* 67(Supplement 2, Part 2):257–87.

————. 1990. Chronic Disease and Disadvantage: The New Politics of HIV Infection. *Journal of Health Politics, Policy and Law* 15:2:341–55. Revised version in *AIDS: The Making of Chronic Disease*. Elizabeth Fee and Daniel M. Fox, eds. Berkeley: University of California Press (1991).

Fox, D. M., P. Day, and R. Klein. 1989. The Power of Professionalism: Policies for AIDS in Britain, Sweden and the United States. *Daedalus* 118:2:93–112.

Grmek, M. 1989. *Histoire du SIDA*. Paris: Playel.

Gross, L. 1989. Personal communication.

Porter, D., and R. Porter. 1988. The Enforcement of Health: The British Debate. In *AIDS: The Burdens of History*. Elizabeth Fee and D. M. Fox, eds. Berkeley: University of California Press.

Silverstein, A. M. 1981. *Pure Politics and Impure Science: The Swine Flu Affair*. Baltimore: Johns Hopkins University Press.

Commentary: Who Calls the Tune?

BARBARA O. DE ZALDUONDO

In the chapter, "Using Social Science to Prevent and Control HIV Infection," Fox makes a number of sobering points for social scientists who aim to improve human health and well-being through their work. He notes, for example, that health policymakers consider and use only a small fraction of the data we produce on the determinants, effects, and social distributions of disease. That is, much of the data that might, or should, provide guidance for improved health policies and programs does not do so. To minimize frustration and wasted time, Fox suggests that behavioral and social scientists recognize the criteria and tactics policymakers use when they acknowledge particular approaches or findings and discounts others. We should inform ourselves about what policymakers want to know about particular health threats or morbidity experiences, such as those connected with HIV infection, and what options for action these policymakers believe they have if they do wish to invest their time and political capital on measures to ameliorate those conditions.

The array of real options, Fox explains, depends heavily on the specific sociocultural and political context in which health policy decisions are to be made. Key structures of this context can be thrown into stark relief, not by reading party platforms or ideological statements, but by examining "who usually does what for and with whom to control and prevent disease" and "how important is prevention and control of the condition in the policy and politics" of the country in question.[1] While behavioral and social scientists may not like the answers revealed in response to these questions, no useful purpose is served by ignoring them. Indeed, if we obdurately neglect these realities, perhaps we deserve the familiar barbs: that behavioral and social scientists respond more to abstract, theoretical agendas and interests than to the practical demands of health promotion. While we may admire the idealism on Don Quixote, he did not, after all, tilt at windmills on public funds. When we fail to address real needs and constraints or fail to detail the practical applications of our work, cries from atop the Ivory Tower— "No one listens to us!"—must be tedious indeed to the more effective advocates of our craft.

Fox's reluctance to extrapolate his analysis from industrialized countries to predictions and/or prescriptions for the health transition in the developing world is well taken. Social and economic models from the one setting often require major overhaul to be valid in the other. Yet some of his arguments, developed through comparison of the United Kingdom, the United States, and Sweden, are all the more compelling in the developing country contexts I know best. For example, Fox explains that policymakers who would like to inform their positions by reviewing the scientific evidence may not find the time to read reams of relevant research results. It is likely that leaders in developing country settings have less staff and time to devote to research and analysis than does the average U.S. member of Congress. Thus, social research interpreted and presented by a trusted advisor as grounds for the wise decision may carry even more weight with harried policymakers in low income countries than in the industrialized West—despite the low market value of wisdom *per se* in the international scientific community. Furthermore, in all countries, allocation of public resources is controlled by the few. While neither political scientist nor historian, I believe it is well established that this process tends to serve the economic interests of the powerful. If so, perhaps compelling arguments that good health is good, and illness is bad, for a nation's economy may do more to increase government investment in health services than any number of passionate humanistic defenses of health as a human right. Rationales stressing economic competitiveness certainly seem to have broadened support for measures to promote education and economic participation of disadvantaged groups—women and ethnic minorities—in the United States.

Other points in Fox's chapter do require recasting when the comparisons and contrasts to be made concern, for example, a Tanzania and a Zaire, or a Canada and a Haiti—that is, when one compares countries governed according to more divergent political philosophies regarding the distribution of the social costs of development. In working democracies, an important amount of accountability and power come from sheer numbers of voters, so the poor—or their advocates—have some influence on public policy. It is probably safe to say that there are few developing countries (Cuba and Nicaragua come to mind) where the disadvantaged majority has anything like the power they have in countries such as the United Kingdom, the United States, and Sweden, where coalitions of the left have a strong voice in the political process. Furthermore, in the United States, the United Kingdom, and Sweden, social scientists can work with the media to influence public opinion in support of medicare and social security for the needy, but in many countries around the world, those who have access to the mass media may not consider the plight of the poor to be their concern.

In this sense, one must reconsider Fox's injunction to social scientists: to see and to engage with the political and economic context that mediates translation of knowledge into policy and praxis. For those who work with the poor and disenfranchised—be it in the industrialized or developing world—scientists and service providers of all disciplines routinely face stark contrasts between the political cultures of their own professions, those of gatekeepers and state representatives, and those of "the people" with and for whom they work. Aside from substantial practical difficulties, moral dilemmas of the most serious proportions may obstruct the path from knowledge to action. Where policymakers or power-holders do not have the welfare of the people at heart, gaining their attention and trust through cultivation of personal relationships, for example, may be out of the question.

The relative paucity of behavioral scientists from, and working in, the developing world is undoubtedly related to this phenomenon. It is predictable that social scientists will find themselves in the role of social critic more often than other professionals, no matter what the government philosophy (Green 1986). Social processes, beliefs, and structures are their subject matter. Scientific research involves empirical work; primary data collection involves contact with the target populations; and the assumptions and stereotypes that, in every culture, are woven into normative ideological rationalizations of self-interest and exploitation tend to fall apart when one works directly with individual members of the caricatured groups. However, in some countries, display or discussion of exploitative norms or institutions is viewed as criticism, and criticism—no matter how well documented and constructively intended—is deemed as or near treason. In such environments, who can afford to perform the function of analyst and critic? Expatriot social scientists may take up this function, being less vulnerable to retribution, but their commentary is likely to be unwelcome, if not inappropriate.[2] It is also likely to be ineffective, unless it is incorporated into the agendas of foreign donor agencies. The latter appear to have a vastly greater impact in defining health and social policy in developing countries than do local health and social scientists. Indeed, perhaps developing country social scientists should target expatriot funding agencies, rather than local policymakers, if they wish to affect health promotion in their own countries.

Thus, if the vista includes the whole range of countries and governments that are approaching the health transition, Fox's parallels between industrialized country and developing country applications of social science become more strained. Some of the actual strategies suggested become unfeasible, or even unethical.

Consider, for example, his reflection that his social science expertise has had the greatest impact when delivered through a personalized, advisory relationship with policymakers. This is not feasible in many developing countries because there are too few local social science experts to go around. Faced with needs for infrastructure and food production, descriptive social science research, like mental health services, has to many countries seemed a luxury they could not afford. In the countries of East and Southern Africa, for example, very few universities have departments of psychology, and anthropology—as distinct from sociology—was actively rejected until quite recently (Herdt 1987). This deficit of university departments implies that incentives for obtaining such training are also curtailed, since the usual job opportunities that await foreign-trained physicians, economists, agronomists, and so forth are unavailable to scholars who invest instead in behavioral science training abroad. Add to this the common concern over social scientists as troublemakers, and one completes the elements of a vicious circle, the regrettable consequences of which have been highlighted by the AIDS pandemic: a deficit of background sociocultural, economic, and health behavior research in developing countries, and a deficit of behavioral and social scientists with the professional training and mandate to correct this gap through research and policy analysis in and for their own countries.

The results of this vicious circle are more complex than one might first imagine. The health transition program is contributing to a global reassessment of the need for social and behavioral science expertise in order to design and evaluate culturally appropriate health education. Cost concerns make short-term technical training attractive; after years of struggle with the "brain drain," funding agencies appear almost to have given up on long-term investments in social science training to the doctoral level. Yet who can compute the costs of the lives that are being lost while countries now attempt to marshal the local behavioral science expertise to design and evaluate interventions for AIDS prevention and care? Will future training budgets reflect recognition of the time and human capital lost while local and foreign physicians and epidemiologists struggled to interpret the distribution and risk factors for HIV infection, and to devise prevention programs in allegedly culture-free, universal biomedical frameworks? Local social scientists might well have been able to see the inappropriateness of early "aerosol" models of HIV transmission, and of culture- and gender-insensitive education and condom distribution programs. Who has calculated the economic losses due to declining tourism in the Caribbean and central and east African countries as a direct result of fear of AIDS, fears that were fueled by inappropriate generalizations and lack of knowledge about the social organization and health behavior of the populations in question (de Zalduondo, Msamanga, and Chen 1989; Farmer 1990)? I imagine these sums would dwarf the costs of staffing and endowing a few professorships in the relevant behavioral sciences in the universities of each affected country.

On the positive side, it should be pointed out that relatively small investments in developing countries, in behavioral and social science research and training, and in catchment area research, can be expected to bring significant returns toward facilitating the health transition. Closer to home, relatively small changes in the orientation of faculty and in the contents of curricula in industrialized country universities could sensitize students and future policymakers to the culture-dependent nature of the social and economic patterns that define the context of health behavior. Presently, industrialized country professors frequently present theories and models in economics, political science, sociology, and psychology as universal, while few of these models and theories have been developed or tested outside western industrial populations and settings. Sensitization to cultural and contextual diversity would focus overdue attention on not only the applied value of empirical data from developing country settings, but also on the advances to basic theory and methods to be expected when members of different cultures approach social theory, health education, political science, and so on with their different biases and transparent assumptions. For example, the cosmopolitan or "western" medical system has much to learn from cultures that do not carve the mind and social context away from the body when it comes to diagnosis, prevention, and management of illness (e.g., Janzen 1978; Kleinman 1986).

Some of the knowledge so urgently needed to guide health policy and planning in the developing world—such as demographic data and descriptive information concerning routine social, economic, and health conditions—is relatively straightforward and simple to collect. What is needed is time, personnel trained in rigorous methods, funds, and the mandate to collect it (Commission on Health Research for Development 1990). In providing this training, time, and funding, however, both the producers and the consumers of such research should take Fox's injunctions to heart and look closely, in advance, at the cultural and structural constraints they will face in promoting the use of these data to improve the public health. Those who work in countries where the government is accountable to the majority, and/or where prevention and control of disease is accorded high priority by the powers that be, may thus more effectively accelerate the uptake of social and behavioral science knowledge in the service of health promotion at home. If we can document consequent benefits in the spheres of economic productivity and/or global prestige and politics, we may also help to change the contextual barriers that constrain the impact of social scientists in other sociopolitical settings.

NOTES

1. Fox found, for example, that despite the public hue and cry surrounding the global pandemic, HIV did not figure prominently at all in the priorities of the participants in his study.

2. This is not to say that industrialized, democratic countries welcome critiques of their political cultures or social agendas, as the McCarthy era and the debate over national health insurance illustrate. De Toqueville may well have been the last foreign social critic to be taken seriously in the United States.

REFERENCES

Commission on Health Research for Development. 1990. *Health Research: Essential Link to Equity in Development*. New York: Oxford University Press.

de Zalduondo, B. O., G. I. Msamanga, and L. C. Chen. 1989. AIDS in Africa: Diversity in the Global Pandemic. *Daedalus* 118:3:165–204.

Farmer, P. 1990. AIDS and Accusation: Haiti, Haitians, and the Geography of Blame. In *Culture and AIDS*. Douglas A. Feldman, ed. New York: Praeger.

Green, E. C. 1986. Themes in the Practice of Development Anthropology. In *Practicing Development Anthropology*. Edward C. Green, ed. Boulder: Westview Press.

Herdt, G. 1987. AIDS and Anthropology. *Anthropology Today* 3:2:1–3.

Janzen, J. M. 1978. *The Quest for Therapy: Medical Pluralism in Lower Zaïre*. Berkeley: University of California Press.

Kleinman, A. 1986. *Social Origins of Distress and Disease: Depression, Neurasthenia, and Pain in Modern China*. New Haven: Yale University Press.

6

The Malaria Transition and the Role of Social Science Research

DONALD R. SAWYER AND DIANA O. SAWYER

INTRODUCTION

A recent initiative of the Rockefeller Foundation provides a perfect statement of the general problem this chapter addresses:

> It has now been recognized that the purely technological approach to health has failed to produce the predicted improvements in health and well-being. One part of the failure lies in the incomplete coverage of the medical services actually delivered, but another part is due to the complexity of the factors affecting susceptibility to and ability to respond to the illness. . . . What is clear is that the reduction of mortality has a major social component as well as a medical one. If we were to understand adequately the social component, and were to employ that knowledge effectively, then we might go far toward achieving the goal of good health for all. (Rockefeller Foundation 1989)

We present here a case study of social science research on malaria. It is based primarily on our own experience in the Amazon region of Brazil, but it also includes some references to other social science research on tropical diseases, especially in Latin America. After briefly describing the malaria transition and resurgence, the chapter focuses on social science research on malaria. It then discusses the theoretical and practical implications of using social science research in the attempt to resume the historical trend of decline in the disease.

MALARIA TRANSITION AND RESURGENCE

Analogous to the demographic transition (Notestein 1945) and the epidemiologic transition (Omran 1971; cited in Omran 1982), as well as more recent proposals suggesting a "health transition" (Findley 1989), one could point to a "malaria transition" in the direction of high to low prevalence or even complete eradication. As was the case in the demographic transition, the change occurred over many decades in the now-developed countries, with relatively primitive medical and vector control technology, and in close relation to broader economic, social, and environmental changes (cf. McKeown 1976). Another parallel with the demographic transition is that since World War II the change in prevalence of malaria in the developing countries has been rapid, occurring over about two decades, and has depended to a large extent on modern health technology imported from developed countries (Caldwell 1976).

A significant difference between the demographic transition and the malaria transition, however, is the fact that the latter has recently changed direction in much of the world. The malaria transition is not just incomplete; it has moved backward. The 1970s saw a resurgence of the disease in many Latin American and Asian countries where it had been brought under control or significant progress toward eradication had been made. While this reversal can be attributed in part to technical factors, that is, resistance to insecticides and drugs, it seems to be due mainly to social, economic, demographic, and environmental forces (WHO 1986).

Brazil provides a good illustration of the reversal in malaria decline (Paula 1986). After national control activities began in the 1940s, malaria decreased from an estimated 6 million cases per year (one-seventh of the population) in 85 percent of the municipalities, to 52,469 officially reported cases in 1970. Seventy-two percent of these were in the Amazon region (Superintendency of Public Health Campaigns 1988:7, Tauil 1984:58). The number of cases has grown steadily ever since, reaching 560,143 in 1990. A million were expected in 1989. While all autochthonous malaria now occurs in the Amazon region, the disease is spreading from new settlement areas to locations where it had formerly been brought under control (Marques 1986b, 1987; Marques, Pinheiro, and Souza 1986).

As a first approximation, malaria in the Amazon can be classified as "frontier malaria." Frontier malaria has distinct characteristics that make it more difficult to control than "stable malaria." There is high vector density and intense exposure to vectors, with significant outdoor transmission. Migrants have low levels of immunity and limited knowledge of the disease. Morbidity is very high and fatality relatively low. Falciparum malaria, much of it drug resistant, predominates. The difficulty of applying conventional control program measures is exacerbated by weak presence of other institutions, little sense of community, and high population mobility as well as political marginality (D. R. Sawyer 1988).

Figure 6.1
Malaria Transition in Frontier Settlements

```
API  :              :                    :
     :              :                    :
3000 :    xxxxx     :                    :
     :  x      xxx  :                    :
     :  x          xxxx                  :
2000 :x            :   xxxxx             :
     :x            :        xxxxxx       :
     :x            :             xxxxxxx
1000 :x            :                    : xxxxxxxx
     :x            :                    :        xxxxxxxxx
     :x            :                    :
   0 :-------------------------------------------------------
     :
Year 0   1    2    3    4    5    6    7    8    9   10   11   12   13
     :              :                    :
     :   Stage 1    :        Stage 2     :    Stage 3
     :   Epidemic   :       Transition   :    Endemic
```

Note: Eradication is not reached within the period considered.

Within this broad category, various specific situations can be distinguished, the most critical of which are new settlements where prevalence is especially high: *garimpos* (small-scale gold mines) and *colonization* (small farming) areas (Marques 1986a; D. R. Sawyer 1988; WHO 1988).

Viewed at the micro level in new agricultural settlements of nonimmune migrants, the malaria transition follows the hypothetical three-stage pattern depicted in Figure 6.1. With conventional control measures, malaria prevalence typically rises rapidly to a peak, which may reach an annual parasite index (API) of 3,000 (three cases of malaria per person per year).[1] It then tapers off gradually over a period of 10 to 15 years. The explanation for this pattern seems to involve the interaction of preventive and curative health activities with ecological and socioeconomic factors. Although some environmental changes, such as flooding behind culverts, may increase malaria, the general trend is to decrease vector density and exposure through clearing of forest, sanitation, and pollution of breeding places (Monte-Mor 1986). In socioeconomic terms, settlers become more established and less mobile, which means that housing, transportation, and communication improve. In turn, immunity increases, making conventional control measures and general health care more feasible and more effective.

The conventional, technological approach to controlling malaria is based on housespraying with DDT, case detection with blood slides, and the distribution of antimalaria drugs. This approach has not been effective, however, in arresting the explosive epidemics of frontier malaria that occur when poor miners and farmers first settle in the Amazon rainforest. The reasons for this are not clear.[2] In the Amazon, in contrast, a program based almost exclusively on DDT and drugs is probably flawed not only in implementation but also in design. That is, the design is probably not entirely appropriate for the present situation of vectors and parasites in new settlements. Operational problems, such as insufficient manpower and material, mean that insecticide coverage is incomplete. As design flaws and operational problems interact, the design cannot be implemented "correctly" in the physical, socioeconomic, and demographic environment of the Amazon. Long distances, warm, humid climates, dense vegetation, high vector density, inadequate roads and transportation infrastructure, the newness of the settlements, the mobility of the population, and the lack of qualified personnel all interfere with the implementation process.

SOCIAL SCIENCE RESEARCH ON MALARIA

What is the present status of social science research on malaria? This section (1) points out the scarcity of existing data, (2) describes briefly the research done at the Center for Development and Regional Planning (CEDEPLAR), and (3) discusses the policy implications of the CEDEPLAR effort.

Scarcity of Social Science Research on Malaria

Scientific researchers have traditionally devoted little attention to the social aspects of malaria. After World War II, the level of interest in this area dropped still further. Investigations that incorporate both social factors and malaria are typically only minimally integrated: Broad studies only touch on malaria, while studies of malaria only touch on social aspects. Few research efforts combine social science in the full sense with a systematic and profound analysis of the disease (Sotiroff-Junker 1978; Sawyer 1986a).

The recent shortage of epidemiological and social research on malaria may be due to epidemiological and social trends themselves. The prevalence of the disease fell in the 1950s and 1960s, becoming limited to peripheral areas. At the same time, there was great faith in the potential of technological breakthroughs (nuclear energy, satellites, vaccines, and antibiotics) for solving economic and social problems. Unfortunately, DDT and chloroquine turned out to be effective "researchicides," as it seemed unnecessary to devote much attention to a disease on its way to eradication.

CEDEPLAR's Research on Malaria

Research carried out at the Center for Development and Regional Planning (CEDEPLAR) of the Federal University of Minas Gerais in Brazil provides an example of the kind of social science research that could contribute to improved control of malaria. CEDEPLAR is a university research and training center that offers postgraduate programs in economics and demography. It became involved in research on malaria during the course of a study of frontier settlement on the Amazon.

The Research

In 1984, sample surveys of 887 households and 385 gold miners were conducted in the region of Tucumã and Ourilândia in Southern Pará, collecting information on epidemiological, socioeconomic, demographic, and environmental variables. Parasitological and serological tests and a small entomological survey were also carried out. The research was conducted in cooperation with SUCAM, the agency of the Brazilian Ministry of Health responsible for the control of endemic diseases.

At SUCAM's request, CEDEPLAR extended the research to Rondônia, organizing a Malaria Perception Survey among settlers selected for the Machadinho Settlement Project. A longitudinal pilot study was begun, with three years of follow-up.

The research team of CEDEPLAR faculty consisted of four economists, two demographers, a sociologist, an architect, and a political scientist. Also involved in the project were scientists at the Oswaldo Cruz Foundation, the René Rachou Research Center, the Department of Parasitology, Federal University of Minas Gerais, SUCAM, and the Center for Population Studies of the University of Campinas. The team spent a year studying malaria through the discussion of basic texts and participation in seminars featuring invited specialists.

The general objective of the research as it was originally defined was as follows: to identify and gauge the relative importance of the various human factors that influence malaria transmission and control in new settlements in the Amazon region. The basic research problem was to discover why, in the high-risk population under field conditions, some groups developed more malaria than others. It followed that once this was known, control measures could be diversified and appropriately targeted. This program would then become more efficient and effective, making it possible to incorporate other sectors and, finally, the population itself, into the overall control effort (WHO 1986).[3]

In July 1985, the team surveyed 358 households in the Machadinho Project. One year later, a second survey covering 818 households was conducted. An analysis of SUCAM's records and small entomological and serological surveys were also carried out by the research team. The regional context of malaria in Machadinho was examined from environmental, economic, demographic, and political perspectives. A historical study of malaria control in Brazil was also undertaken.

The need to find explanations for observed socioeconomic and environmental differences caused the team to return to Machadinho in 1987 to ask new questions about exposure and protection at the individual level. This time 1,050 households in both urban and rural parts of the project were surveyed.

Since it became involved in research on the Amazon, CEDEPLAR has had a close working relationship with SUCAM. The team was invited to provide demographic and sociological consultation on the design of a new program for malaria control in the Amazon basin, a project funded by the World Bank (SUCAM 1988).

Results

The data from the project were analyzed using log-linear models. The principal results of the research in Pará and Rondônia may be summarized as follows.

Very High Morbidity. There were as many as three positive slides per person per year (API of 3,000) in Machadinho. Individuals of both sexes and all ages were affected. However, rates of malaria were higher for men than for women, and higher for adults than for children. A pattern of year-round transmission was identified, with only moderate seasonality.

Strong Economic and Social Impact. Through pervasive, complex, and highly pernicious economic and social effects, malaria contributes to the failure of official settlement projects and to massive rural-urban migration in the Amazon. Small farmers have difficulty replacing disabled labor and so must absorb both direct and indirect loses (Ferreira and Vosti 1987). Malaria contributes to negative selectivity of migrants, the absence of family members, absentee ownership, and low settlement density. It also contributes to high rates of turnover and attrition of those who attempt settlement. Those who remain are often subject to decapitalization and to social polarization between groups that are too poor to leave. Speculators then take advantage of the situation. All of this defeats the social purposes of colonization (cf. Ferreira and Sawyer 1986; Sawyer 1987; Torres 1987; Vosti 1989. See also Bonilla 1987, Mokate 1987).

Strong Socioeconomic, Environmental, and Demographic Differences. Log-linear analysis revealed systematic regularities in the distribution of malaria among categories of socioeconomic, environmental, and demographic variables. The malaria rate for settlers with the most favorable combination of variables (i.e., better housing at a greater distance from the forest, higher income and education, knowledge of the vector, etc.) was as much as six times lower than the rate for those with the least favorable combination. Age and sex differences within households suggest individual differences in exposure outside the home. This impression is confirmed by data from the same surveys. These data focus on specific activities involving different degrees of exposure, for example, clearing, working in the fields, and laundering or bathing in rivers and streams (Fernandez and Sawyer 1986, 1987, 1988, Sawyer and Sawyer 1987; D. O. Sawyer 1988; D. O. Sawyer and D. R. Sawyer 1988).

Outdoor Transmission. Both age and sex differences and the effects of distance from subjects' homes to the forest suggest that exposure to the rainforest environment is responsible for much of the malaria above the level for young children living in houses distant from the forest. This conclusion is supported by entomological data (Sawyer and Sawyer 1987).

Spontaneous Prevention. In the high-risk population, some groups are apparently using effective self-help measures. Whether these take place at the individual or household level, whether they are intentional or incidental, they seem to work under field conditions. Also, prevalence is lower for settlers who have accurate knowledge of the transmission mechanism and who are in a position to apply this knowledge (by virtue of living at a distance from the forest and having economic resources at their disposal).

In sum, the epidemics of frontier malaria seem to be due to a large extent to man's entry into the natural habitat of the vector. The degree of contact with the rainforest explains observed differentials in prevalence. The living conditions and the behavior of the groups with lowest prevalence offer examples that other groups could imitate.

Policy Implications

The results of CEDEPLAR's research point to at least two major implications for policy. First, the existing control strategy should be more closely targeted at the critical points in particular socioeconomic and environmental settings, rather than a shotgun approach. Second, the strategy should be diversified to include not only housespraying, case detection, and treatment, but also low-technology, self-help control emphasizing the participation of the settlers themselves.

The goal in new settlements should be to "cut the peak" of prevalence in the initial epidemic stage and accelerate the transition to lower levels, that is, to flatten the prevalence curve and make it more symmetrical. The results of the research in Tucumã-Ourilândia and Machadinho suggest that relatively modest efforts aimed at expanding and improving the control measures already used by the most malaria-free settlers could reduce prevalence by at least one-third.

Research to date indicates that the following strategies of environmental management, housing improvement, source reduction (control of breeding places), and reduction of exposure to vectors will be useful in achieving this goal:

• Selecting sites for house construction that are at higher elevations and more distant from water;

- Clearing the forest for at least 50 meters around houses;
- Cleaning yards and refraining from planting permanent crops, like coffee, near houses;
- Using wood poles or palm thatch, rather than plastic sheets, to construct the vertical walls of houses or temporary shelters;
- Constructing permanent houses with closure;
- Draining and filling breeding places;
- Facilitating the flow of water in streams;
- Removing vegetation from streams and clearing their edges;
- Digging wells;
- Keeping domestic animals (pigs, cows) near houses;
- Avoiding unnecessary contact with the forest; and
- Avoiding unnecessary contact with water.

A number of additional measures might also be recommended, recognizing that these are not always economically feasible or socially and culturally acceptable. These include the use of bednets, coils, sprays, repellents, protective clothing, screening on doors and windows, and larvicides. Oiling breeding places and staying indoors after dusk are also helpful.

This package of measures is not directed against a particular species or type of behavior (like biting or resting indoors), but rather against a broad spectrum of possible malaria vectors and related behaviors.

Self-help measures such as those recommended here could be evaluated for effectiveness, feasibility, and acceptability, and tested in the field. If they promise to be useful, they could then be promoted through educational programs and community outreach in new settlements of different kinds (Sawyer 1989).

THEORETICAL AND METHODOLOGICAL IMPLICATIONS

We now turn to the question of how social science research can help to reverse the current direction of the malaria transition and reduce the prevalence of malaria to its earlier, lower level in settings like the Amazon. The theoretical and methodological lessons we offer are based on our experience in studying malaria and our familiarity with other social science research on tropical diseases, as well as the growing literature in this area (e.g., Rosenfield 1986; Sevilla-Casas 1987; Hongvivatana 1987; Herrin and Rosenfield 1988).

The Articulation of Two Subcultures: The Social and the Natural Sciences

The mind sets and analytical styles of natural scientists and medical specialists who study malaria are radically different from those of social scientists. Even though both groups claim to be scientists, they might be said to belong to "two cultures," to borrow a term from C. P. Snow (1969). Biological scientists and physicians are accustomed to working with microorganisms or tissues, or at most individual patients, rather than with populations or social systems. At the same time, social science paradigms—social systems, social structures, class, status, power—do not always provide ways of studying health or biological phenomena. This gap is more than a problem of vocabulary. The questions asked, concepts of causation used, units of analysis defined, evidence employed, and criteria of demonstration preferred are all different.

Furthermore, the two subcultures tend to take each other for granted. If, however, the objective is to understand human factors in the transmission, prevention, and cure of disease, each different area of knowledge and competence must have its rightful place. It is not enough to know about social science without knowing about disease. Neither is reading a few basic texts sufficient to make one a social scientist. Finally, professional pride and authority often prevent natural scientists and medical personnel from admitting that social scientists can tell them anything new or important about their own areas of expertise.

It is possible, nonetheless, for the two subcultures to complement each other rather than conflicting. First and foremost, complementarity and communication would be better enhanced if each side simply did better science. Natural science and social science are not focusing on two separate realities, but rather on a single, albeit multifaceted, object: health. Good social science must go beyond the application of ready-made theories or schemes that are often not appropriate for analysis of health problems in contemporary developing countries. The most competent, imaginative, and mature social scientists should be recruited to work on health. Indeed, work on such real-world problems may contribute to the development of the social sciences themselves.

At the same time, there is also a need for good natural science. Too often, supposedly scientific studies are done with no control for confounding factors, no appreciation of bias, inadequate sample sizes, no proper experimental controls, or absolute numbers with no denominators. Nonbiological factors are sometimes totally ignored. Policy decisions that should be based on good natural science often seem to be based on hunches, anecdotes, personal preferences, bureaucratic inertia, or political expediency.

Our research on malaria suggests that in addition to improving social

and natural science research within existing disciplines, there is also a
need for the development of a third, interdisciplinary area capable of
dealing with the ecological and spatial dimensions of health. At least in
the case of a vector-borne disease, it is essential to appreciate the physical
location of the research subjects in relation to breeding, resting, and
biting places, infected individuals, and sources of treatment. These spatial relationships are in constant flux.

Conventional techniques of quantitative analysis do not take into account the changing spatial relationships among cases, but rather treat
them only in terms of their individual characteristics. New tools and
methodologies are needed that use maps, satellite images, spatial variables, community-level variables, and so forth, and involve teams of
geographers, ecologists, architects, urban planners, regional scientists,
and specialists in geographic information systems.

The challenge, however, is not just to combine disciplines that have
tended to work on their own objects of study using their own methods
and techniques. It is also necessary to combine different levels of analysis: environmental, individual, household, community, regional, national, and global. Appropriate conceptual frameworks for articulating
different levels are needed.

Specific Contributions of Social Studies

There are many ways in which social sciences might contribute to a
better understanding of contemporary malaria problems and to improved control. Our experience points especially to the following.

Variability. The variability of malaria across different ecological and
socioeconomic situations is widely recognized. Little is known, however,
about how these types of malaria situations have changed or about the
details of transmission and control in particular kinds of contexts, such
as small-scale mining areas, agricultural settlements, and construction
camps. Better understanding is needed in order to diversify and define
more specific targets for the control strategy (WHO 1986, 1988).

Populations. Demographers and epidemiologists offer a whole kit of
useful tools that could be used by social scientists working on health.
There are lessons to be learned about dealing with entire populations,
not just those who seek treatment. Demographers have developed techniques of making indirect estimates using partial information. Ways have
been found to work with deficient and incomplete data and to deal with
bias. There is considerable experience with analysis of social and economic causes and consequences of biological phenomena (Sawyer 1986c;
Singer 1988).

Field Work. Social scientists, especially anthropologists and sociologists, have a tradition of working in the field—with people—not just in

the laboratory or office. This is the only way to capture and understand the human factors involved.

Behavior and Structure. Social psychological and anthropological approaches may provide insights on malaria-related behavior that could help to facilitate behavior change through intervention (Hongvivatana 1987; Mendez-Dominguez 1987). Popular resistance to DDT, demands for new insecticides, and lack of compliance with drug administration cycles are some of the behavioral issues that must be dealt with, for example, if malaria in the Amazon is to be successfully brought under control.

However, caution should be exercised in attempting to modify behavior. Those responsible for controlling malaria have placed much of the blame for its resurgence in the Amazon in the realm of behavior: widespread migration and mobility, primitive housing, inadequate clothing, close contact with forest and water (Lima 1982; Tauil 1984). It would be unfortunate and misguided to conclude that malaria can only be controlled in the Amazon if and when migration is stopped, houses are screened, water is piped, and settlers wear long trousers and long-sleeved shirts and stay indoors. While these improvements may be desirable, it is also important to recognize that behavior is determined in part by social structure and cannot be changed simply by issuing instructions or, even, improving understanding. Human rights must also be taken into consideration in any attempt to modify behavior. In short, the control strategy must be adapted to the realities of the region, rather than the opposite.

Policy. There has been a clash between overall development policy, which promotes frontier settlement, and more narrowly focused efforts to control the disease, which are seen as the Ministry of Health's sole responsibility. As long as there is no easy technological fix, other government agencies must become involved in the struggle. One of the most important contributions social scientists can make is to show how disease affects development and, therefore, merits public investment in control. This is partly, but not exclusively, a task for economists. As the case of colonization in the Amazon makes clear, development policies are sometimes social policies, and their perverse social effects should be identified (Coimbra 1987).

Community Participation. Community participation and "horizontal integration" (cf. WHO 1983) are much more than a matter of adjusting a control program's structure to new national or international health policies or dividing responsibilities and multiplying available resources. Community participation may also be a technical imperative. The fact of outdoor transmission in the Amazon means that the population itself must become involved in control activities. As SUCAM cannot spray the rainforest, much of this involvement must take the form of self-help.

In the absence of chemical alternatives against the parasites inside human organisms or vectors inside homes, efforts must be directed at vector control outside.

Community participation is not compliance with DDT and drugs, but active control of exposure to vectors. The present, quasi-military vertical structure of some control program is not well suited to working with local populations and other government programs or agencies. Social science could help to overcome the enormous difficulties of (1) defining the concept and content of community participation, (2) dealing with receptivity problems in new areas where "communities" hardly exist, (3) developing approaches that are economically feasible on a large scale, and (4) involving other institutions that are weak on the frontier (D. R. Sawyer and D. O. Sawyer 1988).

PRACTICAL CONSIDERATIONS

There are also practical lessons to be learned about how to achieve the objectives and overcome the obstacles we have outlined. The following partial listing draws on our own experience and on WHO-sponsored meetings in Kuala Lumpur (Reynolds 1986), Salvador (Sawyer 1986b), and Brasília (WHO 1988; Sawyer and Krettli 1988).

In order to bridge the gap between health sciences and social sciences, social scientists must have a basic knowledge of health and health scientists of social sciences. Practitioners of the various disciplines that make up the social sciences (sociologists, economists, political scientists, anthropologists, social psychologists, geographers) and the health sciences (physicians, public health specialists, malariologists, parasitologists, immunologists, entomologists, ecologists, control program personnel) should become more conversant with one another, without losing their own professional competence. The goal is not to create a melting pot but to develop the capability for interaction, dialogue, and collaboration.

Similarly, there is a need for institutional collaboration between developed and developing countries and endemic and nonendemic regions within countries. Such collaboration is necessary in order to integrate advanced technology with a knowledge of the diverse and often puzzling human situations that present new challenges to improved health. So that scientists do not become too esoteric, they must also collaborate with those responsible for preventive and curative health care.

These various collaborative efforts will not occur spontaneously. A sociology of the sociology of health shows us that, being outside the mainstream, the field attracts few students. The low allocation of human financial resources shows that health economics is not a high priority.

Only a major program effort can overcome problems of compartmentalization and marginality and recruit qualified researchers.

A major program effort, however, requires substantial funding. Longitudinal, multidisciplinary field studies involving scientists from institutions in different parts of the world are very expensive. The large numbers of observations required for multivariate analysis also entail high costs. Finally, because it involves marginal subareas within existing disciplines, social science research on malaria requires sufficient funding to make it attractive to researchers who would otherwise tend to gravitate to more conventional topics within established fields.

Since social science research on health is a new area, a major initiative is required to establish collaborative relationships and form a new scientific community. This will entail international and interdisciplinary exchange through scientific meetings, collaborative networks, special publications, and modern communications facilities. Critical reviews of existing knowledge should be made available. Research institutions must be built or strengthened and new personnel trained. Technical assistance, seed money, and small grants (thousands and tens of thousands of dollars) are needed to support the preparation of research proposals and pilot projects that both meet the joint requirements of social and natural science and combine scientific competence with the practical need for improved control. Large amounts (hundreds of thousands of dollars), which are not available in the developing countries, are needed to support the large, long-term, collaborative research projects that will finally provide answers to the complex questions of the health transition. The prerequisite for all of this, of course, is an administrative structure capable of managing such a complex technical and political undertaking both within countries and on a global scale.

CONCLUSION

The reversal of the malaria transition in Latin America and Asia in the last 15 or 20 years occurred in the virtual absence of social science research on the disease and with complete reliance on technological approaches to control. While vaccines, new antimalarial drugs, and new insecticides may help to contain the spread of the disease, it is highly improbable that they will solve the problem in new epidemic areas, which of course pose a threat to all areas where vectors are present. Social science has a large contribution to make. There are clear signs that institutions like the World Health Organization (WHO 1986), the WHO/United Nations Development Program/World Bank Special Programme for Research and Training in Tropical Diseases (Godal 1988), the Brazilian Ministry of Health (SUCAM 1988), the Pan American Health Organization, the Southeast Asia Medical Organization—Tropical Medicine program (Reynolds 1986), and the World Bank are all acutely aware of the need for social science inputs to improve control of tropical diseases. The basic problem is that no one seems to know what to do.

Although in the recent past many health problems were isolated in remote geographical areas or among disadvantaged social groups, increasing global population mobility means that the health problems of specific areas or groups are increasingly becoming global problems. The only way these problems can be solved is through a concerted international effort that combines advanced biomedical and social science tools with village-level knowledge of the complex and mercurial human factors affecting exposure, protection, and treatment. Whether social science research will in fact make a difference in improving or accelerating the health transition in developing countries depends on the improvement of research methodologies, collaboration among disciplines, collaboration between scientists and control programs, and ample and appropriate institutional and financial support.

NOTES

The research on which this chapter is based received support from the Social and Economic Research component of the UNDP/World Bank/WHO Special Programme for Research and Training in Tropical Diseases (Project 840137), the Superintendency of Public Health Campaigns (SUCAM) of Brazil's Ministry of Health, the Collective Health Program of the Financing Agency for Studies and Projects (FINEP) and the National Council for Scientific and Technological Development (CNPq), the International Development Research Centre (Project 3P–84–0098), CNPq's Integrated Program for Endemic Diseases (PIDE VI Processo 40111/85), the Pan American Health Organization, and the World Bank. Nonetheless, the funding was insufficient to carry out the original proposal for a longitudinal, multidisciplinary study with laboratory and entomological components and to complete analysis of the data collected. Analysis is still in progress.

1. A rate of 3,000 was observed in the Machadinho Settlement Project in Ariquemes, Rondônia. At the macro level, these peaks constitute resurgence, or reversal of the previous national downward trend.

2. We do not know why the technical eradication strategy worked in the Northeast and Southeast but not in these situations. Neither is it clear how much of the reduction in malaria in the Northeast and Southeast should be attributed to the control program itself and how much to the effects of "general development": the clearing of forests, greater population density, higher incomes, improvements in sanitation and housing, better education, and expansion of health services. The Northeast and Southeast are vastly different in most of these respects. Important intraregional differences in ecology and levels of de-

velopment also exist. In terms of malaria control, however, the final result was the same in the two regions.

3. Because of funding problems, the project was limited to a pilot study. Emphasis was placed on the development of appropriate methodology, with the goal of providing useful tools for other researchers. The methodological problem was considered to be critical, not only because of the usual difficulties presented by field research in rural areas, but also because research on malaria in the Amazon poses special problems related to the high mobility of the population (Sawyer, Fernandez, and Sawyer 1988).

REFERENCES

Bonilla, C. E. 1987. *Determining Malaria Effects in Rural Colombia.* Paper presented at the Conference on Social and Economic Determinants and Consequences of Malaria and Its Control under Changing Conditions. Sitges, Spain, October 26–28.

Caldwell, J. C. 1976. Toward a Restatement of Demographic Transition Theory. *Population and Development Review* 2:3/4:321–66.

Coimbra, M.A.E.L.S. 1987. Política Pública e Saúde: O Caso da Malária no Brasil. *Análise e Conjuntura* 2:1:72–90.

Fernandez, R. E., and D. O. Sawyer. 1986. Socioeconomic and Environmental Factors Affecting Malaria in an Amazon Frontier Area. In *Economics, Health and Tropical Disease.* A. N. Herrin and P. L. Rosenfield, eds. Manila: University of the Philippines School of Economics.

———. 1987. *Malaria Rates and Fate: A Socio-Economic Study of Malaria among Settlers in a New Settlement Project in Rondonia.* Paper presented at the Conference on Social and Economic Determinants and Consequences of Malaria and Its Control under Changing Conditions. Sitges, Spain, October 26–28.

———. 1988. "Colonização, Malária e Interações: Fatores Sócio-Econômicos e Demográficos da Transmissão de Malária numa Área de Fronteira." Unpublished Manuscript. Belo Horizonte: CEDEPLAR.

Ferreira, A.H.B., and D. R. Sawyer. 1986. Estrutura Produtiva, Migração e Malária: Notas Sobre Duas Áreas Amazônicas. In *População e Saúde: Anais do Seminário Latino-Americano.* Campinas: Editora da Unicamp.

Ferreira, A.H.B., and S. A. Vosti. 1987. "Os Custos da Malária: Considerações Teóricas e Aproximações Empíricas para a Região Tucumã-Ourilândia." Unpublished Manuscript. Belo Horizonte: CEDEPLAR.

Findley, S. E. 1989. *The Health Transition in Developing Countries: Tentative Definition and Processes.* Presentation at the Rockefeller Foundation.

Godal, T. 1988. Address at the Twelfth International Congress for Tropical Medicine and Malaria. Amsterdam, September 18–23.

Herrin, A. L., and R. L. Rosenfield, eds. 1988. *Economics, Health and Tropical Diseases.* Manila: University of the Philippines, School of Economics.

Hongvivatana, T. 1987. *A Conceptual Framework for the Study of Human Behavioral Issues in Malaria.* Paper presented at the Conference on Social and Economic Determinants and Consequences of Malaria and Its Control under Changing Conditions. Sitges, Spain, October 26–28.

Lima, J.T.F. 1982. O Papel da SUCAM na Prevenção e Controle das Doenças no Contexto das Migrações Humanas. In *SUCAM, Doenção e Migração Humana*. Brasília: Centro de Documentação do Ministério da Saúde.

Marques, A. C. 1986a. *Síntese Histórica do Combate à Malária no Brasil e Situação Actual: Evolução da Luta Antipalúdica no Brasil*. Paper presented at the Jornada de Malariologia, Porto Velho, May.

————. 1986b. Migrations and the Dissemination of Malaria in Brazil. *Memórias do Instituto Oswaldo Cruz*, 81, Suppl. II:17–30.

————. 1987. Human Migration and the Spread of Malaria in Brazil. *Parasitology Today* 3:6:166–70.

Marques, A. C., E. A. Pinheiro, and A. G. Souza. 1986. Um Estudo sobre a Dispersária de Casos de Malária no Brasil. *Revista Brasileira de Malariologia e Doenças Tropicais* 38:51–75.

McKeown, T. 1976. *The Modern Rise of Population*. London: Edward Arnold.

Mendez-Dominguez, A. 1987. *Perception of Malaria and Its Influence on Health-Seeking Behavior in Guatemala*. Paper presented at the Conference on Social and Economic Determinants and Consequences of Malaria and Its Control under Changing Conditions. Sitges, Spain, October 26–28.

Mokate, K. M. 1987. *The Intra-Household Resource Allocation Effects of Malaria in Colombia*. Paper presented at the Conference on Social and Economic Determinants and Consequences of Malaria and Its Control under Changing Conditions. Sitges, Spain, October 26–28.

Monte-Mor, R. L. 1986. Malária e Meio-Ambiente na Amazônia Brasileira. In *População e Saúde: Anais do Seminário Latino-Americano*. Campinas: Editora da Unicamp.

Notestein, R. W. 1945. Population: The Long View. In *Food for the World*. T. W. Schultz, ed. Chicago: University of Chicago Press.

Omran, A. R. 1971. The Epidemiological Transition: A Theory of the Epidemiology of Population Change. *Milbank Memorial Fund Quarterly* 49:4(Part 1):509–38.

————. 1982. Epidemiological Transition. In *International Encyclopedia of Population*. J. A. Ross, ed. New York: Free Press.

Paula, J. A. 1986. Passado e Presente de uma Doença Antiga. In *Populaão e Saúde: Anais do Seminário Latino-Americano*. Campinas: Editora da Unicamp.

Reynolds, D. C., ed. 1986. *Social and Economic Research in Tropical Diseases in Southeast Asia with Special Reference to Its Application for Effective Disease Control*. Proceedings of the 29th SEAMEO-TROPMED Seminar, Kuala Lumpur, June. Bangkok: SEAMEO-TROPMED.

Rockefeller Foundation. 1989. *The Health Transition Program: A Proposed Rockefeller Foundation Activity*. New York: Rockefeller Foundation.

Rosenfield, P. L. 1986. Linking Theory with Action: The Use of Social and Economic Research to Improve the Control of Tropical Parasitic Diseases. In *Social and Economic Research in Tropical Diseases in Southeast Asia with Special Reference to Its Application for Effective Disease Control*. D. C. Reynolds, ed. Bangkok: SEAMEO-TROPMED.

Sawyer, D. O. 1988. *Notas sobre Diferenciais Comparativos da Prevalência de Malária em Machadinho, Ariquemes no Anos de 1985 e 1987*. Belo Horizonte: CEDEPLAR.

Sawyer, D. O., and D. R. Sawyer. 1988. *Human Factors in Malaria Prevalence in the Initial Stages of a Settlement Project in Brazil: A Three-Year Follow-Up Study.* Paper presented at the Twelfth International Congress for Tropical Medicine and Malaria. Amsterdam, September 18–23.

Sawyer, D. O., R. E. Fernandez, and D. R. Sawyer. 1988. Socio-Economic and Environmental Differentials of Malaria Prevalence: Notes on Methodology. In *Economics, Health and Tropical Disease.* A. N. Herrin and P. L. Rosenfield, eds. Manila: University of the Philippines, School of Economics.

Sawyer, D. R. 1986a. The Potential Contribution of Social Research to Control of Malaria in Brazil. *Memórias do Instituto Oswaldo Cruz* 81:(Suppl. II):31–37.

———. 1986b. *Informe Final sobre la Reunión de una Red sobre Ciencias Sociales y Malaria, Salvador, Bahia, Brasil, 9–10 de Agosto de 1986.* Belo Horizonte: CEDEPLAR.

———. 1986c. "Demography and the Epidemiology of Malaria: Notes on Similarities and Applications." Unpublished Manuscript. Belo Horizonte: CEDEPLAR.

———. 1987. *Economic and Social Consequences of Changing Patterns of Malaria in New Colonization Projects in Brazil.* Paper presented at the Conference on Social and Economic Determinants and Consequences of Malaria and Its Control under Changing Conditions. Sitges, Spain, October 26–28.

———. 1988. *Frontier Malaria in the Amazon Region of Brazil: Types of Malaria Situations and Some Implications for Control.* Paper presented at the PAHO/WHO/TDR Technical Consultation on Research in Support of Malaria Control in the Amazon. Brasilia, April 28–30.

———. 1989. *Malaria on the Amazon Frontier: Integrated Participation for Control of Malaria in New Agricultural Settlements.* Belo Horizonte: CEDEPLAR.

Sawyer, D. R., and A. U. Krettli. 1988. *Pesquisa em Malária no Brasil: Notas sobre Prioridades.* Paper prepared for the National Research Council of Brazil.

Sawyer, D. R., and D. O. Sawyer. 1988. *Community Participation in Malaria Control.* Paper presented at the Twelfth International Congress for Tropical Medicine and Malaria. Amsterdam, September 18–23.

Sawyer, D. R., and D. O. Sawyer, coords. 1987. *Malaria on the Amazon Frontier: Economic and Social Aspects of Transmission and Control.* Belo Horizonte: CEDEPLAR.

Sevilla-Casas, E. 1987. *The Study of Social and Economic Determinants of Malaria: Theoretical and Methodological Issues.* Paper presented at the Conference on Social and Economic Determinants and Consequences of Malaria and Its Control under Changing Conditions. Sitges, Spain, October 26–28.

Singer, B. 1988. *New Approaches to Research in the Social Sciences.* Unpublished manuscript. New Haven: Yale University.

Snow, C. P., 1969. *The Two Cultures and a Second Look.* Cambridge: Cambridge University Press.

Sotiroff-Junker, J. 1978. *A Bibliography on the Behavioural, Social, and Economic Aspects of Malaria and Its Control.* Geneva: WHO.

Superintendency of Public Health Campaigns. 1988. *Programa de Controle da Malária na Bacia Amazonica.* Brasília: SUCAM.

Tauil, P. L. 1984. Malária: Agrava-se o Quadro da Doença no Brasil. *Ciencia Hoje* 2:12:58–64.

Torres, H. G. 1987. *Desistência e Substituição de Colonos em Projetos de Colonizaão de Rondônia: Um Estudo de Caso.* Belo Horizonte: CEDEPLAR.

Vosti, S. A. 1989. *Land Use Patterns in the Humid Tropics: A Case Study of the Machadinho Colonization Project in Northwest Brazil.* Washington, D.C.: International Food Policy Research Institute.

World Health Organization. 1983. *Community Participation in Tropical Disease Control: Social and Economic Research Issues.* Geneva: WHO.

————. 1986. *WHO Expert Committee on Malaria.* 18th Report. Geneva: WHO.

————. 1988. *Report on a Technical Consultation on Research in Support of Malaria Control in the Amazon Basin*, Brasília. Geneva: WHO.

Commentary: Old Themes and New Directions in Malaria Studies

ELIAS SEVILLA-CASAS

The choice of malaria as one of the case studies to be discussed here is not coincidental. The health transition discussion is in some ways a return to old fields in public health that have been kept fallow for several decades.

Malaria is still the greatest killer in the tropics, where as a chronic disease it has successfully resisted many ingenious attempts at control. As we prepare to celebrate a century of successes and failures in the effort to control malaria, and as we look forward to new technological breakthroughs in synthetic vaccines, it is convenient to look back and learn from history.

Malariology made a serious strategic error in placing too much confidence in the technological advance of residual insecticides during the eradication campaign that ended in 1978. It is instructive to recall the warning issued by the Malaria Commission of the League of Nations in 1927: "The history of anti-malarial campaigns is chiefly a record of exaggerated expectations followed sooner or later by disappointment and abandonment of the work" (quoted in Jeffrey 1976).

Although in the pre-eradicationist era social scientists were not formally considered to be participants in programs of malaria control, it is clear that this statement refers essentially to a problem of human behavior and organization. Nowadays, social science is considered a high priority in malaria work (WHO 1988a). The failure of the eradication campaign has taught us, among other lessons, that the study of the behavior of Homo sapiens is as important as the study of the behavior of mosquitoes and parasites in the fight against malaria (Gillet 1985; Kitron 1987).

A number of other damaging errors were made in the eradicationist era. One was stopping research. Another was forgetting that the "social problems," as P. F. Russell called them in 1943, were not going to be solved with purely technological methods (Russell 1943). Losing the capability of moving across a vast array of measures of control, a flexibility that was characteristic of the "old" malariology, was a third unfortunate error made during the eradicationist campaign.

The Rockefeller Foundation deserves credit for supporting many of the pioneering efforts to develop flexible and holistic approaches to control (Harrison 1978). The names of Drs. Hackett, Soper, Logan, and Russell are associated with the many lessons we are now learning again about malaria control. The formal introduction of social science research into programs of malaria control represents the continuation of a trend following an unfortunate, 35-year hiatus. Happily, social science disciplines appear to be mature enough to successfully meet the challenge.

"The Malaria Transition and the Role of Social Science Research," by Donald and Diana Oya Sawyer, presents an overview of the authors' research on malaria in the Amazon Valley. The discussion is set within the context of the revival of old themes and offers a good example of the maturity of our disciplines. Indeed, these authors use the entire armamentarium of social science research to explicitly address the complexity of human behavior. This complexity is illustrated by the fact that man has on the one hand contributed to the maintenance and spread of malaria in the Amazon Valley, while at the same time organizing efforts to stop the spread of the disease and reduce incidence to tolerable levels. The result is a contradiction between the man-made expansion of malaria on the frontier of colonization and the unsuccessful man-made organization for its control. Many social scientists have addressed this contradiction (Barbira-Scazzocchio 1980, WHO 1988b), which seems to lie at the heart of Brazilian society. In general terms (Zeleny 1985), it reflects the inadequate adjustment of an artificial social organization and structure, one designed to bring about the control of a disease, to the spontaneous social orders of the peasant colonies. This adjustment seems to be a crucial area of study for modern interdisciplinary research (Allen 1985).

The Sawyers are studying a "malarious ecotone," that is, a transitional zone between two ecological communities, one of which has well-established relations between man, mosquitoes, and parasites, and one of which does not (Pianka 1983). The term "ecological community" is used here to refer to a network in which populations of several species, including human groups, interact in a determinate habitat (Reed 1988; Schoener 1986). The high instability initially observed in the malarious ecotone becomes more settled with the passage of time. This is what the Sawyers refer to as the "malaria transition."

The terminus ad quem of the transition is not, however, equilibrium, as the commonly used (WHO 1988c) term "stable malarias" may suggest. Rather, it is a condition of near-equilibrium (DeAngelis and Waterhouse 1987; Maurer 1987) in human populations that are faced with a series of socioecological constraints. Malaria is only one of a number of life problems these populations have to solve.

Under "settled" conditions, malaria fluctuates between being more or less of a priority. Other diseases and life demands may at any given time compete successfully for the attention and resources of the local people (Najera 1979). However, under ecotonic conditions, the terminus a quo of the transition, the situation is different. In these circumstances, morbidity and mortality caused by malaria are always very much on people's minds (WHO 1988c).

One of the most important contributions the Sawyers have made to malaria studies is their empirical handling of the various phenomenological manifestations of the disease—as mere infection, as detected parasitaemias, as a clinical complex of bodily signs, and as illness or sickness. There is no need to dwell here on the distinctions among these, as they have already been discussed in the social scientific literature (Kleinman 1987; Young 1982). Project reports from the Amazon describe the problems involved in differentiating among manifestations of malaria under field conditions. Interdisciplinary work in serology, parasitology, clinical medicine, and anthropology is urgently needed to define and measure malaria in its various forms.

To illustrate both the broad range of social science questions the health transition raises and the problems involved in attempting to define malaria, I will briefly present some comparative material. The following is taken from the field studies we are currently carrying out on the Pacific coast of Colombia (Sevilla-Casas 1988).

Consider two contrasting situations. On the Pacific coast we have found the frequencies of the phenomenological manifestations of malaria to be arranged in the form of a pyramid. The pyramid is similar in shape to the frequency pyramids used to describe the hierarchical arrangements of trophic levels in ecology (Odum 1971). That is, in a given population (100 percent) the rate of malaria infection, as detected by serology, is approximately 80 percent. Only a very low proportion, however (approximately 3 percent) show clinical signs that are locally recognized as warranting a change in activities. The functional definition of malaria illness as a condition necessitating a change in the routines of daily life is extremely important, as it represents a broader conception of risk than the "objective risk" measured by epidemiologists (Slovic 1987). This broader conception includes both objective risk and its subjective perception and assessment. The subjective perception and evaluation of risk is the key to understanding people's decisions to act to prevent or treat malaria.

In the Amazonian ecotonic situation, in contrast, the multilayered manifestation of malaric entities has a rectangular form. The Sawyers' data indicate a 70 to 90 percent rate of infection and a similar rate of parasitaemias, clinical manifestations, and reported illness.

The difference between the pyramid and the rectangular forms of the phenomenology of malaria in settled and ecotonic situations stems primarily, although not exclusively, from differences in the immunological make-ups of the two populations. Two additional, related points pose interesting questions for social scientists. First, immunological response in human populations is highly influenced by neurological, psychological, and sociological factors, about which very little is known. Second, a routine question for future interdisciplinary research on malaria should be, "Which manifestation of malaria is being referred to?" A report from WHO (1986) indicates, for example, that sub-Saharan Africa's image as an endemic area for malaria is substantially changed when the disease is defined as a clinical entity rather than as a rate of generic infection.

The Sawyers would no doubt agree that the definition of malaria as an illness that is experienced and managed by local people is extremely important in both ecotonic and settled conditions. In providing numerous practical, conceptual, and methodological insights, their work breaks new ground for the study of malaria from this perspective.

REFERENCES

Allen, P. M. 1985. Towards a New Science of Complex Systems. In *The Science and Praxis of Complexity: Contributions to the Symposium Held at Montpellier, France, 9–11 May, 1984.* United Nations University, ed. Tokyo: United Nations University.

Barbira-Scazzocchio, F., ed. 1980. *Land, People and Planning in Contemporary Amazonia.* Occasional Publication No. 3. Cambridge: Cambridge University Centre of Latin American Studies.

DeAngelis, D. L., and J. C. Waterhouse. 1987. Equilibrium and Non-Equilibrium Concepts in Ecological Models. *Ecological Monographs* 57:1–21.

Gillet, J. D. 1985. The Behavior of *Homo Sapiens*, the Forgotten Factor in the Transmission of Tropical Disease. *Transactions of the Royal Society of Tropical Medicine and Hygiene* 79:12–20.

Harrison, G. 1978. *Mosquitoes, Malaria, and Man: A History of the Hostilities since 1880.* New York: E. P. Dutton.

Jeffrey, C. M. 1976. Malaria Control in the Twentieth Century. *American Journal of Tropical Medicine and Hygiene* 25:366.

Kitron, U. 1987. Malaria, Agriculture and Development: Lessons from Past Campaigns. *International Journal of Health Services* 17:295–326.

Kleinman, A. 1987. *The Conceptual Basis for the Study of Illness Perception and Behavior in Tropical Diseases.* Paper presented at the Conference on Social and Economic Determinants and Consequences of Malaria and Its Control under Changing Conditions. Sitges, Spain, October 26–28.

Maurer, B. A. 1987. Scaling of Biological Community Structure: A Systems Approach to Community Complexity. *Journal of Theoretical Biology* 127:97–110.

Najera, J. A. 1979. A Suggested Approach to Malaria Control and to the Methodology Applicable in Different Epidemiological Situations Based on the Experience in the Americas. *Bulletin of the PanAmerican Health Organization* 13:223–34.

Odum, E. P. 1971. *Fundamentals of Ecology.* New York: Harper and Row.

Pianka, E. R. 1983. *Evolutionary Ecology.* New York: Harper and Row.

Reed, E. S. 1988. The Afrodances of the Animate Environment: Social Science from the Ecological Point of View. In *What Is an Animal?* T. Ingold, ed. London: Unwin Hyman.

Russell, P. F. 1943. Malaria and Its Influence on World Health. *Bulletin of the New York Academy of Medicine* 19:599–630.

Schoener, T. W. 1986. Overview: Kinds of Ecological Communities—Ecology Becomes Pluralistic. In *Community Ecology.* J. M. Diamond and T. J. Case, eds. New York: Harper and Row.

Sevilla-Casas, E. 1988. *Human Aspects of Seasonality, Mobility, and Malaria in the Naya River Basin of Colombia.* Final Report of a project supported by the UNDP/WORLD BANK/WHO Special Programme for Research and Training in Tropical Diseases. Cali: Universidad del Valle.

Slovic, P. 1987. Perception of Risk. *Science* 236:280–85.

World Health Organization. 1986. *WHO Expert Committee on Malaria: Eighteenth Report.* WHO Technical Report Series 735. Geneva: WHO.

———. 1988a. *Priorities for Social and Economic Research in Onchocerciasis, Malaria, Methodology and Health Policy.* Report of the Fifth Meeting of the Scientific Working Group of Social and Economic Research. UNDP/WORLD BANK/WHO Special Programme for Research and Training in Tropical Diseases. Document TDR/SER/SWG(5)/88/3. Geneva: WHO.

———. 1988b. *Report on a Technical Consultation on Research in Support of Malaria Control in the Amazon Basin.* UNDP/WORLD BANK/WHO Speical Programme for Research and Training in Tropical Diseases. Document TDR/FIELDMAL/SC/AMAZ/88/3. Geneva:WHO.

———. 1988c. Malaria Diagnosis: Memorandum from a WHO Meeting. *Bulletin of the World Health Organization* 66:575–94.

Young, A. 1982. *The Anthropologies of Illness and Sickness.* Vol. 11, *Annual Review of Anthropology.* Palo Alto: Annual Reviews, Inc.

Zeleny, M. 1985. Spontaneous Social Orders. In *The Science and Praxis of Complexity: Contributions to the Symposium Held at Montpellier, France, 9–11 May, 1984.* United Nations University, ed. Tokyo: United Nations University.

7

Dietary Management of Diarrhea in Peru

GUILLERMO LOPEZ DE ROMANA, HILARY M. CREED, MARY FUKUMOTO, ENRIQUE R. JACOBY, AND SOFIA S. MADRID

BACKGROUND

Several community-based studies from developing countries have demonstrated that poor infant feeding weaning practices, along with frequent infections, are the major determinants of growth inhibiting and malnutrition. This is true even where food availability at the household level is adequate (Black, Brown, and Becker 1974; Martorell Habicht, Yarbrough, Lechtig, Klein, and Western 1975; Mata 1978; Rowland, Cole, and Whitehead 1977; Rowland, Rowland, and Cole 1988). It is therefore reasonable to expect that improved nutritional management during and after illnesses should result in better nutritional status of children in the affected populations.

Diarrheal disease control programs have generally recognized this relationship and have, therefore, attempted to promote appropriate dietary management in the context of oral rehydration therapy programs. However, the educational messages that have been developed are generally nonspecific, simply promoting continued breast-feeding and continued feeding of the usual diet. Specific directions as to what types and quantities of foods should be offered, and how long and how frequently such improved dietary regimens should be implemented for each illness episode, are lacking. Without such specific guidelines, it is difficult for mothers to apply current programmatic recommendations.

At the same time, the kinds of specific messages we are advocating must be compatible with cultural, socioeconomic, and ecological realities. They must address the recommended nutritional requirements of healthy children as well as any additional requirements imposed by the presence of disease. Thus, local information is needed in order to define existing feeding practices in relation to diarrhea and identify possible improvements.

In Peru, as in many developing countries, high rates of infant mortality are due principally to poor nutritional status and high incidence of infectious disease. A National Nutrition and Health Survey (Encuesta Nacional de Nutricion y Salud, 1984) showed that 38.5 percent of children under three years of age were moderately or severely malnourished, the rural populations of the highlands showing the highest malnutrition levels. A longitudinal study of children aged up to one year carried out in one of the *pueblos jovenes* (shanty towns) of Lima revealed the incidence of diarrhea to be as high as 10 episodes per child, per year (López de Romaña, Brown, Black, and Kanahiro 1989). A survey based on a representative sample of one of the departments of Peru (Ancash) yielded similar results (Lanata and Black 1986).

The Dietary Management of Diarrhea (DMD) Program was established to design, implement, and assess a programmatic intervention to reduce or eliminate the adverse nutritional consequences of childhood diarrhea in a region of Peru with high prevalences of malnutrition and diarrheal diseases. The program is administered by the Instituto de Investigacion Nutricional (IIN) in collaboration with the Ministry of Health and the Johns Hopkins University.

BACKGROUND RESEARCH

Management of the research and intervention activities was the responsibility of an interdisciplinary team composed of two pediatricians, several nutritionists, an anthropologist, and a number of a public health specialists. A national advisory committee was also convened to oversee the project and to review preliminary results and future plans as the work developed.

The programmatic activities were undertaken in the Callejon de Huaylas, an Andean valley of the central highlands. Approximately 100,000 people live in the valley, which is located about 150 km northeast of Lima. Most inhabitants of this area depend on agricultural activities for their livelihood. The major crops produced are wheat, potatoes, maize, and a variety of garden vegetables.

In order to plan the DMD intervention, baseline information was obtained on the following: (1) nutritional status of children in the target population, (2) current feeding practices for infants and young children (both during diarrhea and when free from illness), (3) the foods habitually consumed by these children, (4) other foods available in the valley, (5) the cost and seasonal availability of these foods, and (6) cultural attitudes regarding the use of these foods in children's diets.

Observations of the dietary intake of a small number of children were completed in order to quantify the amounts of foods and nutrients consumed by these children at three time points: (1) during episodes of diarrhea, (2) during recuperation, and (3) after recovery. This background research was completed over the course of one year before the pilot intervention program was begun.

At the same time that these issues were being examined, information was also collected on potential avenues for disseminating the dietary recommendations developed by the project. Both traditional methods of communication and mass media were considered. Finally, health professionals were interviewed as a way of assessing the current beliefs, recommendations, and therapeutic practices of the professional community.

Detailed information on the anthropometric status of children in the target area was available to the project from the National Nutrition and Health Survey, or ENNSA. The results of the survey indicated that the rates of low height-for-age (defined as less than -2 Z scores) among children under six years of age were about 42 percent in urban areas and 64 percent in rural areas of the central highlands. These rates were among the highest in the country. Except for information about nutritional status and breast-feeding practices, no data on dietary habits were available from the ENNSA survey.

In light of this, a number of studies were conducted by the DMD project team in order to obtain the necessary information. As a first step, background information on infant feeding practices, local definitions of illness, child care activities, and women's work roles was collected using rapid ethnographic assessments (Bentley, Pelto, Schumann, Strauss, Oni, Adegbola, De la Peña, and Brown 1988). A sample survey was then completed using a representative cluster sampling technique. The families of approximately 2,500 children under three years of age were interviewed as part of this study. Forty-three percent of the respondents were from urban areas and 57 percent were from rural areas.

Information on the age at which other foods and liquids were introduced into the diet was obtained in the survey in two ways. First, a list of commonly available foods was prepared on the basis of data from the ethnographic assessments. Care-givers were then presented with the list and asked to indicate how frequently each food was consumed by the children under their charge. Second, 24-hour dietary histories detailing food consumption for the day before the survey were elicited. Care-givers were also questioned about the diets of their children during diarrhea.

The results of the survey indicated that diarrhea was extremely common. Point prevalence rates reached 20 percent for children from 6 to 23 months. Data on feeding practices showed nearly universal use of breast-feeding. The median age for weaning was 21 months (Figure 7.1).

Figure 7.1
Percentage of Children Currently Breast-Feeding, by Age and Residence,
Callejón de Huaylas, Perú

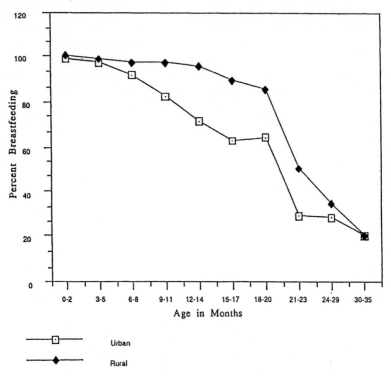

Despite the high prevalence and adequate duration of breast-feeding, the survey data showed that other liquids were added to the diet at an unnecessarily early age.

Twenty percent of infants less than one month old received other liquids in addition to breast milk. At five months, this figure rises to approximately 80 percent (Figure 7.2). In each instance, infants in urban areas were more likely to receive other liquids than those in rural areas. The early introduction of nonhuman milks was also common, particularly in urban areas (Figure 7.3). Thus, exclusive breast-feeding was practiced by fewer mothers than anticipated. The majority of infants began to receive solid foods by five months of age. Almost all infants were receiving solids by nine months (Figure 7.4).

The 24-hour recall histories showed that the foods most commonly consumed by children over six months were wheat, potato, rice, noodles, bread, and maize. The legumes most often consumed were peas

Figure 7.2
Percentage of Young Infants Receiving Other Liquids in Addition to Breast Milk, by Age and Residence, Callejón de Huaylas, Perú

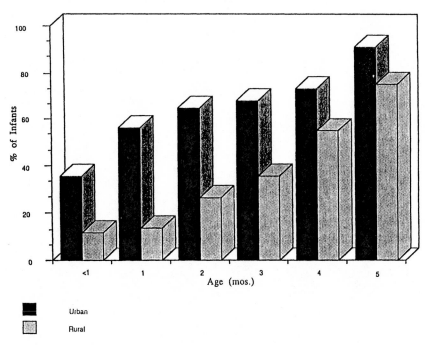

and fava beans. Typically, these foods were prepared as soups. All of these foods are produced locally in the valley except rice and noodles.

Almost all mothers reported that they continued breast-feeding during episodes of diarrhea. Some mothers, however, noted that they stopped feeding other (nonhuman) milks and solid foods. Further probing revealed that the reason for this "interrupted feeding" was almost always the child's unwillingness to eat, not the mother's unwillingness to feed. It appeared that except for nonhuman milks, no particular food was withdrawn from children's diets during diarrhea.

Observational studies were also completed in one rural village in order to measure the amounts of food and nutrients consumed by children during and after diarrhea. Structured behavioral observations were conducted by dietary workers to determine whether changes in feeding practices or in children's appetites could explain observed differences in food and nutrient intake.

Home surveillance of diarrheal disease was carried out by field workers living in the community under study. That is, on the date following identification of a new episode of diarrhea, a dietary worker measured

Figure 7.3
Percentage of Young Infants Receiving Nonhuman Milk, by Age and
Residence, Callejón de Huaylas, Perú

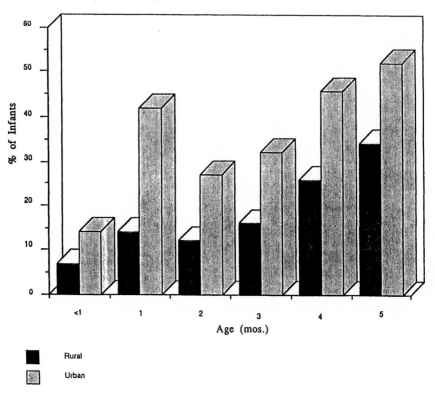

all foods and breast milk consumed by the child during a full day (12 hours) of observations. This procedure was completed for 45 children aged 3 to 36 months on alternate days during diarrhea, early convalescence, and for several days following recovery. The children consumed approximately 75 kcal/kg/day during diarrhea, 81 kcal/kg/day during convalescence, and 84 kcal/kg/day on the day after recovery. There was no evidence of food withholding during diarrhea, although foods and liquids of lower energy density were offered more frequently.

Energy intake was not increased during convalescence to make up for the insufficient intake during diarrhea. Even in healthy periods, intakes were substantially lower than recommended amounts. For these reasons, it was concluded that the most appropriate intervention strategy was the development and promotion of nutritionally enhanced weaning foods that could be considered appropriate for use during diarrhea. Because of the many demands on their time, it was considered unlikely

Figure 7.4
Percentage of Infants Receiving Solid Foods, by Age and Residence,
Callejón de Huaylas, Perú

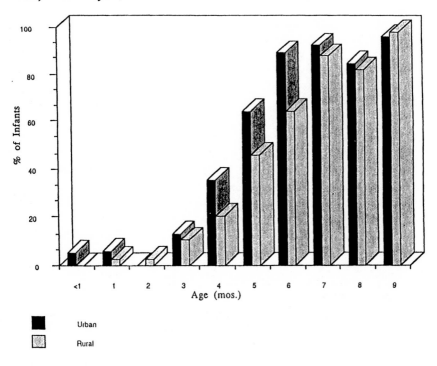

that mothers would be able to feed their children more than the usual three times per day.

Additional studies were then conducted to identify nutritionally appropriate low cost foods that would be available to families in this region. Food cost data were obtained from quarterly market surveys. The costs per unit of energy of selected nutrients was computed. At the same time, information obtained from the sample survey already described was analyzed to identify appropriate channels for the dissemination of feeding recommendations.

The survey showed that approximately 60 percent of the inhabitants of the valley spoke Spanish, while 30 percent spoke Quechua. The remaining 10 percent spoke a dialect that combined the two languages. This meant that it would be necessary to prepare messages in both Spanish and Quechua in order to assure complete coverage of the zone, including the rural areas. Since the vast majority of households had radios that were in daily use, audio programming was selected as the primary medium of communication. More than 90 percent of households had at least one person who was able to read, meaning that written materials could be used to support the diffusion of radio messages.

The survey data also revealed that between 70 and 80 percent of parents traveled outside of their communities each week, most often to the market. This meant the marketplace could be a site of face-to-face product demonstrations.

THE INTERVENTION

Several major decisions that together defined an intervention strategy were made on the basis of these research results. The first decision was to develop an improved weaning food (i.e., higher in calories, protein, and other nutrients) that could be used for the treatment of diarrhea. Second, it was decided that information about these recipes would be disseminated through radio messages and face-to-face demonstrations in community-based organizations and rural marketplaces. The radio messages were intended to promote awareness, and the demonstrations would provide detailed information on methods of preparation. The third decision was to train health professionals in the preparation and use of these recipes, so that they would actively and enthusiastically support the intervention plan.

The first step in carrying out the intervention was to develop prototype recipes using foods that were low in cost, locally available, and culturally acceptable. The recipes were intended to combine foods in ways that would produce a nutritionally adequate diet. To insure their ultimate acceptability, the recipes were developed in consultation with mothers using a series of "recipe trials." The trials were conducted in several rural and urban communities. They involved presenting low cost, readily available foods to groups of mothers, who were then asked to collaborate in formulating one or more recipes using combinations of these foods. The energy densities of the resulting dishes, the time required for preparation, and the cost of the mixed diet were then evaluated. The mothers' comments on the various products were also recorded. The most frequent preparations were soups or puddings composed of wheat-legume mixtures, or stews or purees prepared from potato and other ingredients.

A few mothers, however, made *Sanco*. Sanco is traditionally prepared from pork fat, toasted wheat flour, and sugar or salt. It is a fairly dry "snack food" that is used as an alternative to bread. During the recipe trials, Sanco was prepared with the addition of grated carrot and flours prepared from toasted pea or fava bean. The final recipe had an energy density of approximately 200 calories/100 g and could be prepared in less than 10 minutes. This was the highest calorie density and the shortest preparation time of all the recipes identified. Further study indicated that this product was highly acceptable to infants and children with diarrhea.

In order to test the efficacy of this product in the treatment of diarrhea, clinical trials were conducted among hospitalized children. One group of children received the Sanco product, while a second group received a commercially available, lactose-free formula diet. Severity of diarrhea (fecal excretion rates), duration of illness, amount of food consumed, and net absorption of macronutrients were then measured in both groups.

Preliminary results from these studies indicated similar responses to the diets and similar rates of fecal excretion in the two patient samples. Duration of illness was shorter, however, among those patients who received the product formulated from locally available foods. These results, derived from the second phase of research, were used to plan educational messages and materials promoting the use of this recipe for children during and after diarrhea.

A product name, "Sanquito," was adopted to indicate that the traditional Sanco had been adapted especially for young children. In order to persuade mothers of the usefulness of the product, cultural data were collected on local concepts of health and the appropriate feeding of children. These concepts were used to motivate mothers to prepare Sanquito.

Because of the popularity of traditional folk music, a well-known local folksinger was recruited to record a song describing the preparation and use of Sanquito. A photograph of the singer feeding a child Sanquito was reproduced on a calendar for distribution to mothers who participated in training sessions. This calendar, which was intended to be placed on the wall of the home, also included pictures of the Sanquito recipe. A flipchart was also prepared to demonstrate the steps involved in the preparation of Sanquito. All of these educational materials were pretested and revised prior to final printing.

Cooking demonstrations were conducted in two settings. First, nutritionists from several voluntary agencies and the regional office of the Ministry of Health were trained to teach members of local mothers' clubs how to prepare Sanquito. Following the training sessions, each nutritionist received a flipchart and a set of calendars to be distributed to participating mothers.

Other supporting materials included "Radio Novelas," or radio soap operas, that included themes incorporating the use of Sanquito. Finally, public services messages were aired periodically on the radio in order to promote the use of the project recipe.

After the first round of mothers' clubs demonstrations was completed, nutritionists from the study team conducted demonstrations in major marketplaces in the valley. A troupe of "street actors" was recruited to prepare promotional skits about the use of Sanquito. Preparation of the recipe was demonstrated while these skits were being performed.

Before the educational intervention was begun, coordinating meetings were held with the implementing agencies. Professional training seminars were held on two occasions during the project.

A newsletter was prepared by the project team and printed and distributed periodically by the Ministry of Health. The newsletter included reviews of recent publications from the international scientific literature as well as results of project activities in Peru. Eventually, the project newsletter was incorporated into a similar newsletter distributed by the Child Survival Program of the Ministry of Health.

Finally, promotional materials were prepared for health professionals in the area. These included prescription pads printed with the Sanquito recipe and diarrhea treatment recommendations, and "advertising materials" provided by the distributors of commercial drugs. These efforts were intended to educate health professionals about the objectives and activities of the project and to solicit their collaboration.

EVALUATION

The educational intervention was formally initiated in March 1988, and it continued for six months. Several types of evaluation exercises were carried out during the final stages of the project and after it was completed. First, health professionals were interviewed to determine whether they had received the promotional materials and used them in their clinical practice. Second, a sample survey of approximately 350 households was conducted to assess the members' knowledge of Sanquito and their trial and adoption rates. Third, in-depth interviews were conducted with mothers to examine their perceptions of Sanquito and their reasons for adopting or not adopting the product.

Preliminary results of these evaluations indicated that 82 percent of the population had heard about Sanquito. The principal channel of communication for this purpose was the radio.

Twenty-five percent of respondents (N = 533) who had learned about Sanquito through a face-to-face demonstration, plus other channels of communication (such as radio messages), had prepared the recipe within four months of the launching of the project. Only 10 percent of respondents who had not participated in a face-to-face demonstration had used the product.

The two principal reasons given by mothers for not preparing the recipe were (1) they did not known how to do it, or (2) their children had not had diarrhea. Mothers who had participated in a face-to-face demonstration were less likely to say that they did not know how to prepare the product. Ninety-five percent of the respondents who had prepared Sanquito said they would like to continue using it.

LESSONS LEARNED

This project was one of the first major efforts to develop feeding interventions to combat diarrheal disease. The objectives of the project were therefore not only to implement programmatic activities but also to assess the value of various applied research methods for program development. For this reason the range of research activities was greater than would normally be required by diarrheal disease control or primary health care programs.

Much of the information required for program development may already exist in many countries. For example, information on children's nutritional status, feeding practices, dietary intake, and treatment of diarrhea may be available. In these cases, background research activities could start with recipe trials. When sufficient background information is not available, a great deal of useful material can be obtained from rapidly completed anthropological assessment.

Comparisons of data obtained from survey, direct observation, and abbreviated anthropological techniques indicated that similar conclusions could be drawn from each research method. This suggests that the use of anthropological techniques alone would be appropriate for applied programs if the requisite skills and expertise were available.

Two aspects of this effort deserve special mention. First, the interdisciplinary collaboration that took place as part of the project was critical to its success. Constant communication among experts in a variety of disciplines was necessary to provide a holistic appreciation of the many issues that affect child feeding practices. Moreover, frequent communication among the individuals who carried out the background research and those who used the resulting data to develop programmatic messages was essential to keep the research focused on the ultimate programmatic objectives.

A second important feature of the project was the interactive nature of the research activities. Following each phase of data collection in the field, a formal meeting of the entire interdisciplinary team was convened to review the results of the completed studies and to plan the next phase of investigation. This enabled the research team to identify new areas of importance at various stages of the process and then to obtain relevant information on these areas.

NOTE

Many individuals assisted in the development of the concepts and techniques described here. Of particular importance were the contributions of Kenneth H.

Brown, Sandra Huffman, Margaret Bentley, and Steven Esrey from the Johns Hopkins University, and Cecilia Verzosa from the Academy for Educational Development. This work was supported by the Office of Nutrition, Agency for International Development, Cooperative Agreement No. DAN–1010—A, entitled "Dietary Management of Diarrhea (DMD) Project." Additional support was provided by the local USAID mission in Lima.

REFERENCES

Bentley, M. E., G. H. Pelto, D. Schumann, W. Strauss, G. A. Oni, C. Adegbola, M. De la Peña, and K. H. Brown. 1988. Rapid Ethnographic Assessment: Applications in a Diarrhea Management Program. *Social Science and Medicine* 27:107–16.

Black, R. E., K. H. Brown, and S. Becker. 1974. Effects of Diarrhea Associated with Specific Enteropathogens on the Growth of Children in Rural Bangladesh. *Pediatrics* 73:799–895.

Encuesta Nacional de Nutricion y Salud. 1984. *Direccion General de Censos y Encuestas.* Lima, Peru: Enero, Survey published as a book in 1986.

Lanata, C., and R. E. Black. 1986. *Development of Survey Methodology to Assess Childhood Health Status and Service Utilization. Annual Report.* Lima, Peru: Board of Science and Technology for International Development, National Academy of Sciences.

López de Romaña, G., K. H. Brown, R. E. Black, and H. Kanashiro. 1989. Longitudinal Studies of Infectious Diseases and Physical Growth in Infants in Huáscar, an Underprivileged Peri-Urban Community of Lima, Perú. *American Journal of Epidemiology* 129:769–84.

Martorell, R., J. P. Habicht, C. Yarbrough, A. Lechtig, R. E. Klein, and K. A. Western. 1975. Acute Morbidity and Physical Growth in Rural Guatemalan Children. *American Journal of Diseases of Children* 129:1296–1301.

Mata, L. J. 1978. *The Children of Santa Maria Canque: A Prospective Field Study of Health and Growth.* Cambridge, Mass.: MIT Press.

Rowland, M.G.M., S.G.J. Rowland, and T. J. Cole. 1988. Impact of Infection on the Growth of Children from 0 to 2 Years in an Urban West African Community. *American Journal of Clinical Nutrition* 47:134–38.

Rowland, M.G.M., T. J. Cole, and R. G. Whitehead. 1977. A Quantitative Study into the Role of Infection in Determining Nutritional Status in Gambian Village Children. *British Journal of Nutrition* 37:441–50.

8

Assessment of Health Program Performance to Improve Management: Utilization of Lot Quality Assurance Sampling to Increase Immunization Coverage in Peru

CLAUDIO F. LANATA, ROBERT E. BLACK,
GEORGE STROH, JR., AND HILDA GONZALES

The health status of a community can be improved by actions at two levels: the community itself and health services. In this chapter we concentrate on the level of health services to see if a community's health status can be improved by helping health managers optimize the performance of health programs.

Monitoring and evaluation are two important tools used in the management of health programs. Monitoring focuses on the process of health care delivery, while evaluation determines a program's outcome and impact. Because of the cost and difficulty of evaluating impact, most management efforts are limited to monitoring, that is, measuring process and some outcome indicators. In some cases, health officials use process indicators (e.g., number of vaccine doses given) to estimate outcomes (e.g., immunization coverage). There is a need to develop methods that can measure outcome rapidly and easily, in order to make this information useful for improving health programs.

Health surveys have frequently been used to measure both the outcome and the impact of health programs. Traditional survey methods, however, are costly, requiring full-time personnel and lengthy periods of data collection and analysis. Furthermore, there is considerable lag time between the completion of the survey and the availability of the results. This makes it difficult for officials in charge of health programs to use the information in decisionmaking. Finally, these health surveys provide information at a regional or national level, rather than at the level of small population units. This means that their results are not helpful in directing supervisory activities to areas with the greatest need.

Lot Quality Assurance Sampling (LQAS) (Dodge and Romig 1959;

Rienke 1988) is a survey technique developed in industry for use in quality control. The technique involves identifying one or more small population units (lots) assigned to separate health teams. Small random samples are then selected in each lot to determine which lots conform (or fail to conform) to a given standard of health program performance. This allows health planners to direct supervision and redistribute resources to the most needed areas, thereby maximizing the chances of improving overall program performance.

Because only small samples are required, the LQAS survey can be completed within hours by a single supervisor in each lot, as part of other supervisory activities. More than one health program can be evaluated and lots can be sampled as frequently as needed. Another advantage of this method is that results from all lots sampled can be combined to provide a precise estimate of overall program performance for larger population units or regions.

The research reported here represents the first attempt to evaluate Lot Quality Assurance Sampling for use in health programs.

OVERVIEW OF THE LQAS METHOD

The LQAS method may be summarized as follows (Lanata, Stroh, Black, and Gonzales 1990). First, one or more lots are demarcated in each health unit. The lots are defined as geographical areas that the health program considers sufficiently distinct to justify separate evaluation and program action, even if they are in the same larger health unit. A complete list of households (census) is then compiled for each lot. One or two key indicators, such as immunization coverage or proportion of diarrhea cases treated with oral rehydration solutions, are selected for each health program to be evaluated.

Previous observations of program performance are used to define two levels of expected performance for each key indicator: satisfactory and unsatisfactory. A series of operating characteristic (OC) curves (Dodge and Romig 1959; U.S. Department of Agriculture 1966) or sample size tables (Lemeshow and Stroh 1988, 1989) are then used to select a sample size for a particular sample scheme to be used. The sample size is selected to minimize errors of classification, that is, mistaken acceptance of a lot as satisfactory (type I error), or mistaken rejection of a lot as unsatisfactory (type II error).

A sampling scheme is then selected. A sampling scheme defines the minimum number of individuals to be assessed and the maximum number of "defects," that is, individuals who do not meet the satisfactory level of expected performance specified for each health indicator permissible for acceptance within the sample (Rienke 1988).

If multiple health indicators are used, the final sample size will be the

Table 8.1
Utilization of Lot Quality Assurance Sampling in Evaluating the Performance Level of Health Programs in Twelve Health Zones (Lots) in Canto Grande, Lima, Peru, September 1984

Program Indicators	Satisfactory-Unsatisfactory Performance Level (%)	No. of Lots Rejected	Overall Performance Level (%)
ORS knowledge	50 - 10	0	78 (86-70)*
ORS use	50 - 10	5	32 (41-23)
Prenatal care	40 - 10	1	66 (75-57)
Immunization card	80 - 30	4	70 (78-62)
Immunization coverage	80 - 30	4	64 (73-55)

* percentage (95% confidence intervals)

largest sample calculated for any single indicator. A random selection of households equal to the needed sample size is then made from the census list. One individual is identified in each designated (or adjacent) household. The lot is classified as acceptable for each indicator if the number of defects is not greater than the number defined by the sample scheme.

PILOT FIELD TESTS OF THE LQAS METHOD

Field Test 1. The first step in field testing the LQAS method was to conduct a multipurpose survey in a peri-urban community in Lima, Peru. The survey was designed to evaluate the performance of the diarrheal disease control program, the prenatal care program, and the immunization program in that area. Two indicators were selected for the diarrheal disease program: (1) whether mothers knew about oral rehydration solutions (ORS), and (2) whether mothers had used ORS during the most recent diarrheal episode in a child under five years of age.

For the prenatal care program, the indicator selected was whether a pregnant woman had attended a prenatal care clinic at least once. Two indicators were selected for the immunization program: (1) whether a child aged 3 to 14 months had an immunization card, and (2) whether that child had had all of the immunizations recommended for his or her age.

For each program indicator, several OC curves were used to select sample schemes in which specific (satisfactory and unsatisfactory) expected performance levels were utilized (Table 8.1). Because previous information on the indicators was not available, the judgment of local health officials was used to define levels of expected performance. The sample size was nine, and the total number of permissible defects was two or three, depending on the performance levels selected for the various indicators.

Twelve areas (lots) were demarcated using information from the census tracts. A team of four health workers conducted the survey in the 12 lots, consisting of a total population of 85,929 individuals, in one week. Five lots were rejected for their level of ORS use, but none for ORS knowledge. One lot was rejected because of the low coverage of the prenatal care program, and four lots were rejected for their level of immunization coverage and availability of immunization cards (Table 8.1). Overall weighted estimates for the level of performance on each indicator were calculated for the area.

This field test demonstrates that the LQAS technique can be used to evaluate multiple health programs. The lots identified as unacceptable became the focus of additional supervisory activities.

Field Test 2. As a second field test, we decided to evaluate the change in immunization coverage following a nationwide immunization campaign conducted by the Peruvian Ministry of Health in October 1984. The campaign was pronounced successful by health officials on the basis of the number of vaccine dosages delivered relative to the size of the targeted population, as estimated by the 1981 census.

An LQAS survey was carried out one week after the termination of the campaign (Lanata, Stroh, and Black 1988). Anticipating an increase in immunization coverage, we designated 90 percent coverage as the satisfactory level of expected performance and 65 percent as the unsatisfactory level. A sample size of 14 children per lot with a maximum of two defects permissible for acceptance was selected as the sampling scheme.

All 12 lots were rejected. The combined estimate of coverage for the entire area was 62 percent (95 percent confidence interval of 55 to 69 percent). This was not different from the estimate obtained before the immunization campaign (see Table 8.1).

To discover why no improvement in postcampaign immunization coverage was found, we visited all of the health posts in the area and reviewed their immunization records. Several problems in the way the campaign was carried out were identified as a result. For example, only 20 percent of the vaccine doses were given to children under one year old. Because much of the vaccine was used for children up to age 15, several immunization centers reported shortages of vaccine and syringes. This resulted in failure to vaccinate 20 to 50 percent of young children who visited the immunization post. Thus the real increase in immunization coverage in children under one year appeared to be less than 4 percent, a proportion undetectable given the sample size used in the LQAS survey.

EVALUATING THE LQAS METHOD'S CAPACITY TO IMPROVE MANAGEMENT

Given the positive results of the field pilot testing of the LQAS method, the next step was to determine whether local health officials in charge of an immunization program would use the LQAS results to modify their planning of subsequent initiatives, thereby improving overall immunization coverage. To investigate this, we decided to use the LQAS method to evaluate immunization coverage in areas outside Lima, in the Peruvian Andes mountains. The sites chosen for the evaluation were the city of Huaraz, located at 3,200 meters above sea level, and several nearby rural and small urban communities located up to 4,500 meters above sea level (Lanata, Stroh, Black, and Gonzales 1990).

All health units in charge of immunization in the study area were included. Twelve population areas (lots) were then selected. Six of these were in urban and six in rural areas. One health unit had only one population lot; another had three lots; the others had two lots each. A total of 16,373 households with 81,031 inhabitants were enumerated in the household census conducted in each lot. All of the households identified in each lot were listed in geographic order. This listing was then used as a sampling frame.

A small baseline random sample survey was conducted during the completion of the census in September 1986. The survey found 72 percent of the children aged one to four years in the study area to have been immunized with three doses of diphtheria, pertussis, and tetanus vaccine (DPT), oral poliomyelitis vaccine (OPV), and one dose of measles vaccine (95 percent confidence interval, 59 to 85 percent).

Three nationwide immunization campaigns, to be conducted during one weekend each in October, November, and December of 1986, were planned by the Ministry of Health. The objective was to achieve complete immunization of 80 percent of all children aged one to four years. Instructions were given to mobilize all available resources, including community volunteers, to attain this goal. National radio, television, and newspaper coverage were directed toward the campaign, which was called "VAN 86." Every health post had specifically designed posters inviting people to immunize their children as part of the effort. Finally, most health units sent their immunization teams to distant communities to inform the population of the dates of the campaign and to request that children be brought to central areas for immunization.

An LQAS survey was conducted one week after the first massive immunization effort. On the basis of data from the baseline survey, the level of acceptable coverage was defined as complete immunization (all scheduled doses of DPT, OPV, and measles) for 90 percent of children aged one to four years. The unacceptable level was set at 60 percent. Using a double sampling scheme, an initial sample size of seven was selected. If all of the children in the sample were fully immunized, the lot was accepted. If three children were found to be less than fully vaccinated, the lot was considered unacceptable. If one or two children in the first sample were found to be less than fully immunized, a second sample of up to eight children was drawn. The children in the second sample were then surveyed one by one until three children in the two samples were found to be less than fully immunized (and the lot considered unacceptable), or until the second sample was finished (and the lot considered accepted).

A double sampling scheme was selected for this survey because it would have been theoretically advantageous if most lots could have been classified using only the first sample. It proved difficult to carry out, however, especially in sparsely populated and remote rural areas, where the surveyors had to return to difficult-to-reach areas that they had already visited in order to draw the second sample. Only five of the 12 lots were classified as acceptable according to the LQAS survey conducted after the first nationwide immunization effort (Table 8.2). The weighted estimate of overall population coverage was 78 percent (95 percent confidence interval: 69 to 87 percent).

One week before the second stage of the campaign, health officials were informed of the LQAS survey results. They reacted on the one hand with satisfaction, because the estimate of overall coverage was close to the targeted level, and on the other with confusion. Their confusion stemmed from the fact that the areas they considered to have the highest coverage were the lots rejected in the LQAS survey, while the lots thought to have the lowest coverage were accepted. The officials agreed to direct increased attention to two health units whose two constituent lots had been defined as unacceptable. Most of the volunteer workers were sent to help these units.

The unacceptability of rural lots was found to be due in part to the fact that the immunization teams had to leave their central posts to travel to these areas during working hours, thus arriving at a time when most mothers and children were out working in the fields. To remedy this, the Ministry of Health authorized the immunization teams to travel the day before and to spend the night in the rural areas, in order to be ready to vaccinate during the early morning hours. As compensation, team members received equivalent time off the following week.

A second LQAS survey, using the same definitions of acceptable and unacceptable performance (90 percent and 60 percent, respec-

Table 8.2
Application of Lot Quality Assurance Sampling (LQAS) to Monitoring Immunization Coverage in Twelve Population Areas (Lots) Covered by Six Health Units in Three Massive Immunization Campaigns, Huaraz, Ancash, Peru, October–December 1986

Lot No.	Health Unit No.	Lot Character	No. of Children 1-4 yrs old	1st LQAS Lot Rejected	2nd LQAS Lot Rejected	3rd LQAS Lot Rejected
1	1	Urban	66			
2	1	Rural	288	Yes		Yes
3	2	Urban	403	Yes	Yes	
4	2	Rural	433	Yes	Yes	Yes
5	3	Rural	356			Yes
6	4	Urban	1125			Yes
7	4	Urban	1376			
8	4	Rural	1045	Yes		
9	5	Urban	584	Yes	Yes	Yes
10	5	Rural	630	Yes	Yes	
11	6	Urban	705	Yes		Yes
12	6	Rural	522	Und*	Yes	Yes

* Undetermined: field team did not complete sample scheme.

tively), was carried out after the second stage of the campaign. Because of the difficulties presented by the double sampling scheme, a single sampling scheme was substituted in the second survey. The single scheme consisted of a sample size of 13 or 14 children (depending on the lot target population size) and a maximum permissible number of two defects (children aged one to four less than fully immunized) per lot.

Seven of the 12 lots were classified as acceptable in the second survey (see Table 8.2). Two health units that had had both their lots rejected in the initial survey had both lots rejected a second time. Only three health units had a lot rejected. The weighted estimate of coverage in the overall area increased to 82 percent (95 percent confidence interval: 76 to 88 percent).

The results of the second LQAS survey were given to the health authorities at the time they were analyzing the official immunization coverage statistics. These statistics had been prepared according to instructions from the central headquarters of the Ministry of Health in Lima. The official statistics were based on the number of vaccine doses given and on the 1981 census-based population estimates projected for 1986 for each of the health units. They showed lower coverage levels than the levels estimated by the LQAS for overall coverage.

Some health officers were concerned about an apparent discrepancy in reporting. The official statistics showed the urban lots of the fourth health unit to have 50 percent coverage, whereas the immunization team insisted that not a single unvaccinated child was revealed in their door-to-door search. These officers were relieved when the LQAS data indicated that coverage in these urban areas was in fact high, and that overall coverage had improved since the previous survey. They also noted that two health units with previously rejected lots and a third unit with one rural lot rejected were the only units with problem areas.

Several decisions were made by the health officials after they received the LQAS survey results.

First, a decision to carry out further investigation of the three problematic health units revealed management difficulties involving the head nurses in charge of distributing resources and the immunization team. The three head nurses were removed from their posts and replaced.

Second, a decision was made not to use official estimates, because they contained an error in the assessment of the target population. Rather, it was decided to focus efforts and resources on the areas with lower coverage levels as demonstrated by LQAS.

A third LQAS survey was carried out one week after the final stage of the immunization campaign. Because an improvement in the level of immunization coverage was expected, acceptable and unacceptable levels of expected performance were reset at 95 percent and 70 percent, respectively. This change resulted in an increased single sample size of 18 to 27 and a maximum number of children not fully immunized of two to three per lot.

The survey showed six lots to be acceptable. Three of the lots that were rejected were also rejected in the prior LQAS surveys. Additional time was needed to complete this survey due to the larger sample size. Overall immunization coverage was estimated at 88 percent (95 percent confidence interval: 84–92 percent).

While showing an overall improvement in immunization coverage, the results of the third LQAS survey were surprising in that lots previously classified as acceptable were rejected. The only explanation found for this trend was that during the third immunization campaign, the Ministry of Health delivered measles vaccine in multiple dose vials instead of the single dose vials used in the previous two campaigns. This meant that some vaccination teams had a shortage of measles vaccine while others had an excess.

As a result of this finding, area health officials decided to conduct a fourth massive door-to-door campaign, even though it had not been planned for the nation. They expressed their appreciation of the LQAS studies and their desire to have the methodology available both in the health area and in more distant areas where measles outbreaks were occurring.

DISCUSSION AND CONCLUSION

Field testing of the LQAS has documented two ways in which the methodology may be useful. First, it offers a method for monitoring health programs, such as the Peruvian immunization program. Second, it generates timely and precise information that health officials can use to improve program performance. Despite an inadequate level of financial and logistical support, the health system (with the assistance of volunteers) was able to use data from LQAS surveys to raise the level of immunization coverage in six health areas in the mountains of Peru from 72 percent to 88 percent in three months.

The LQAS contributed to this achievement in a number of ways. First, several key discussions occurred in response to the information provided by the LQAS surveys that made it possible to improve planning for subsequent stages of the campaign. Second, several specific decisions were made that would not have been possible had the LQAS data not been available. They were (1) allowing immunization teams to travel in advance to distant areas, (2) replacing the nurses in charge of coordinating immunization activities in three health units, and (3) redistributing human and logistical support to the most needed area. Finally, the information from the LQAS revealed to health officials the severe limitations of using a method of estimating immunization coverage that is based on the number of vaccine doses administered and the population estimates for various geographical areas.

In addition to providing information to health officials, the LQAS methodology contributed to improving the level of immunization coverage by motivating immunization teams, who were aware that their performance was being monitored by independent observers. The survey results created competition among immunization teams and produced a sense of accomplishment when a particular team's area was judged to have good coverage.

It is important to note in this regard that on the whole, the level of motivation of the immunization teams appeared to be excellent. The teams had always felt that official estimates of the target population assigned to each health unit were incorrect. Many had even conducted previous annual censuses to assist them in planning health program activities. This valuable information was never used, however, by the central health planners because they did not trust it. As a result, some health units satisfied themselves with the minimum required effort, even in areas where the population estimates were lower than the real number of children.

The motivation of some health units suffered, however, because they received consistently poor evaluations from the central health office even though they made efforts to find unimmunized children (who did not really exist). The LQAS results provided the information necessary for the accurate recognition of good and bad performance, while the methodology itself offered a tool for improving communication and understanding between the central health officials and the local health units.

Unfortunately, several obstacles to making the LQAS methodology available to health planners still exist. The primary obstacle is the complexity of the processes of (1) calculating sample sizes and allowable numbers of defects and (2) interpreting the survey results. These processes must be simplified if the methodology is to become accessible to health planners.

Another obstacle is the need for a random sample, which requires a good population sampling frame. Frequent community censuses are necessary to keep such a sampling frame up to date.

The need for a highly committed supervisory team is another obstacle to the successful implementation of the LQAS methodology by health planners. The temptation to simplify the survey process by omitting actual visits to selected households when significant travel is involved is very strong. Also, lack of transportation, which is still a considerable problem for many health programs in developing countries, means that supervisory teams will be less likely to carry out these surveys as often as they should.

Our hope is that the LQAS methodology will be made more accessible to health officials in the near future and that it will then be used frequently to monitor health programs and enhance the usefulness of supervisory activities. Health planners and health teams can improve their performance in implementing health programs by using tools like LQAS to generate timely and accurate information about small health areas.

NOTE

Financial support for this project was provided in part by the U.S. Academy of Sciences/National Research Council by means of a grant from the U.S. Agency for International Development. The authors wish to thank the director, Dr. Jose Alamo-Palacios, and the personnel of the Ministry of Health, Ancash Departmental Health Unit, for their assistance and participation in this project. All correspondence should be addressed to Claudio F. Lanata, M.D., Instituto de Investigacion Nutricional (I.I.N.), A.P. 18–0191, Lima 18, Peru.

REFERENCES

Dodge, H. F., and H. G. Romig. 1959. *Sampling Inspection Tables: Single and Double Sampling.* New York: John Wiley and Sons.

Lanata, C. F., G. Stroh, Jr., and R. E. Black. 1988. Lot Quality Assurance Sampling in Health Monitoring. *Lancet* i:122–23.

Lanata, C. F., G. Stroh, Jr., R. E. Black, and H. Gonzales. 1990. Usefulness of Lot Quality Assurance Sampling in Monitoring and Improving Immunization Coverage. *Int. J. Epidemiol* 19:1086–90.

Lemeshow, S., and G. Stroh, Jr. 1988. *Sampling Techniques for Evaluating Health Parameters in Developing Countries.* Board on Science and Technology for International Development (BOSTID), National Research Council. Washington, D.C.: National Academy Press, pp. 1–38.

———. 1989. Quality Assurance Sampling for Evaluating Health Parameters in Developing Countries. *Survey Methodology* 15:71–81.

Rienke, W. A. 1988. *Industrial Sampling Plans: Prospects for Public Health Applications.* Occasional Paper No. 2 Institute for International Programs, The Johns Hopkins University School of Hygiene and Public Health. Baltimore: Johns Hopkins Printing Services, pp. 1–36.

U.S. Department of Agriculture, Consumer and Marketing Service. 1966. *Accuracy in Attribute Sampling: A Guide for Inspection Personnel.* Washington, D.C.: U.S. Department of Health, Education, and Welfare, Public Health Service.

Commentary: Targeted Interventions for Immunization and Diarrhea Management

CARLA MAKHLOUF OBERMEYER

Chapter 7 and 8 present the results of two creative intervention projects that used a combination of approaches to deal with infant and child health problems. Lot Quality Assurance Sampling (LQAS), as described by Lanata, is a method inspired by industrial quality control that elaborates on the evaluation methods of the Expanded Program of Immunization (EPI) to insure the efficient operation of vaccination programs. The diarrhea intervention program described by Romana integrates the work of a multidisciplinary team with the inputs of mothers in order to improve the management of weanling diarrhea. Both chapters describe the ways in which a health intervention can be fine-tuned to be more effective in the context in which it is applied.

The interventions used to deal with infant diarrhea are different in design from those that aim at improving vaccination coverage. The diseases that are the target of immunization programs (usually polio, diphtheria, pertussis, tetanus, and measles) are caused by specific entities, and once the optimal sequence of vaccines has been administered, the intervention is deemed successful in granting lifelong immunity. That is why immunization can be carried out using mobile teams and is often a vertical program administered by the central government, sometimes in collaboration with an international agency. What we call diarrhea, by contrast, is the result of infection by a multitude of enteric pathogens (bacteria, viruses, and parasites). It may also accompany infections that are not specific to the gastrointestinal tract, such as malaria, pneumonia, streptococcal infection, or measles. In most cases, no lifelong immunity is conferred. Diarrhea management therefore requires a more continuous intervention. The constant need for services is obvious when we remember that, on average, children under five living in less developed countries suffer two to 10 episodes of diarrhea per year. The two chapters describe the ways in which two different health programs can be made to run more efficiently.

The fundamental differences between diarrhea management and vaccination programs, however, should not obscure the fact that in both cases, the major obstacles to improved health for infants and children are found in the poverty and socioeconomic conditions that increase the chances of contamination and infection and make the cost of seeking preventive and curative care too high for many families. This issue seems central, especially in the context of a discussion of the cultural, social, and behavioral aspects of health. But neither of the two chapters addresses it. The extent to which social science constituted a significant ingredient in their respective "recipes" for solving problems is limited. Social science is totally absent from the Lanata chapter. It makes a timid appearance in the Romana chapter, which reports that the suggestions of social scientists were sought to improve the social marketing of the weaning food. The programs described by Lanata and Romana represent ingenious solutions to the technical complexities of the situations they have to deal with. Despite their different foci, the authors have in common the choice of a single targeted intervention. Lanata's chapter is most concerned with improving the efficiency of the procedure used to test vaccination coverage, while Romana's describes the efforts deployed to improve diarrhea at one specific time in the life of the infant. In their dedication to refining the technical aspects of a health intervention, they are good examples of successful programs. However, in the context of a broader discussion aimed at understanding the health transition, they appear as instances of what Henry Mosley calls "involution"[1]: the tendency to focus on internal functioning rather than on determinants and consequences.

Social science tells us that targeted interventions that do not deal with the root causes of ill health can have only a limited impact. Hence the constant dilemma: Should resources be directed only toward those limited technical aspects of the problems that one can deal with in a cost-effective way, or should they be used to address the fundamental determinants of health problems? Vertical targeted interventions may be more effective, but it is in part because their goals have been narrowly defined and their internal functioning has received more attention than their overall impact. It may even be that in the context of the current debt crisis being experienced by many less developed nations, it is precisely the combination of effective targeted interventions and worsening economic conditions that accounts in part for the phenomenon of improved mortality accompanied by worsening morbidity that has been observed in recent years. It would be unfortunate if the contribution of social sciences to the health transition were limited to working within the confines of targeted interventions without questioning how these "solutions" come to be defined, how relevant they are to the sociocultural context, and what their broader consequences are.

NOTE

1. This term is borrowed from Clifford Geertz's anthropological study of the social and economic history of an Indonesian town.

PART III
SOCIAL SCIENCE RESEARCH AND THE IMPROVEMENT OF HEALTH

9

Health and Development: What Can Research Contribute?

NANCY BIRDSALL

INTRODUCTION

In this chapter I discuss, all too briefly, the state of research on relations between health and economic development. The discussion is far from inclusive in coverage of the issues,[1] let alone of the large and growing literature, and is heavily focused on the contribution of economists. My purpose is limited and specific. It is to provide the necessary background to address the question: How has such research contributed, indirectly if not directly, to improved health[2] of populations in the developing world? And how might such research contribute in the future?

I divide the discussion into two parts: the effects of development on health (or, more broadly, the determinants of health status, including nonhealth factors that change with development such as income, education, the relative price of food, transport, communications, and so forth); and the effects of health on development.

This chapter began around a simple set of notes for an oral presentation and grew in length based on many useful comments from readers. Perhaps because of this incremental approach, the discussion is not explicitly linked to any underlying theory or set of assumptions. A few notes on assumptions here will, I hope, at least inform the reader about my prejudices. Central assumptions include:

- Health is produced by households, along with a number of other valued goods, as a function of the resources the household has and the constraints and opportunities it faces; the process of development affects health in part by changing those resources, constraints, and opportunities.

• Development depends in part on investment in human capital, including health; improvement in health of individuals is thus likely to influence the amount and process of development.

• Both health and other aspects of development are affected by public policies. Public policies are affected by many political, economic, and social interests; policies are also and can also be affected be better information and thus by better research.

Finally, the contribution of research can be and is considered in this chapter from both a positive and a normative point of view. Research can help us understand the links between health and development in a positive sense; given that understanding, it can help us in formulating improved health policy to foster development, and improved development policy to foster better health, either directly or indirectly.

THE EFFECTS OF DEVELOPMENT ON HEALTH

State of the Art

Statistical analyses of the determinants of life expectancy and other measures of mortality across nations, mostly by demographers, provide insight into the effects of development (defined here as improvements in the material welfare of the reference population) on individual health. For example, Preston (1980) found that per capita income and adult literacy, but not a measure of calorie availability, were closely associated with life expectancy both in 1940 and 1970. However, only half the increase in life expectancy over the intervening 30 years could be explained by changes in the values of those variables. The rest was apparently attributable to changes in public health technology, general improvements in transportation and communication, and—possibly— changes in the distribution of income or access to health services that were favorable to health. Wheeler (1980) similarly found an increase in life expectancy between 1960 and 1970 that could not be fully explained by such variables as per capita income, adult literacy, population per doctor, and population per nurse.

These cross-national studies establish associations between various indicators of development and health, but they cannot inform us about whether more development actually causes better health (either on average for entire communities or for those individuals whose higher income or better education is measured as "more development"). An example of our ignorance of the causal sequence emerges indirectly from the studies just noted: Although per capita income is associated with or correlated with low mortality (poorer countries having generally higher mortality),[3] high per capita income is by no means a prerequisite to countries achieving low mortality and thus better levels of health. This lesson is aptly captured in a set of studies entitled *Good Health at Low Cost*, which consists of case studies of a group of countries and regions that have achieved low mortality despite low per capita incomes, including China, Sri Lanka, the state of Kerala in India, and (at somewhat higher incomes) Cuba and Costa Rica (Halstead, Walsh, and Warren 1985).[4]

Because there are no internationally comparable measures of morbidity, there have been no cross-national studies of the correlates of morbidity (independent of mortality). In fact, since the available measures of mortality heavily reflect infant and child, as opposed to adult, mortality, it is fair to say that existing studies across countries provide little insight into the effects of development on adult mortality or on morbidity at any age (that does not result in death in the short run). I will return to this general issue later in my discussion.

Compared to studies at the national level, studies at the individual and household level have greater potential for revealing underlying behavioral and causal relationships. There is a growing literature on the determinants of health status at the household level, made possible by the increasing availability of household data for developing countries that include such measures of health status as infant and child mortality and (more rarely) anthropometric measures. Behrman and Deolalikar (1988) provide an extensive and careful review of these studies. They conclude that at the household level it is difficult to document that higher income improves health.[5] This result may reflect the high correlation of income with other variables that are generally included in such analyses, such as education; and the much greater tendency of such variables as education to reflect past behavior and investments that heavily influence current health. Or it may be, as seems to be true at the national level, that other factors (most notably, mother's education[6]) are more important determinants of the health of household members. Behrman and Deolalikar also conclude that there is little evidence that higher prices, be they for health services, for health goods such as drugs, or for food (and thus nutrition, an important input to good health), contribute to poor health.

Thus, the two variables that economists might assume would influence health, income, and prices appear to explain little at the household level. Why these poor results? It may be that community-level variables, such as climate, exposure to disease, and the quality of available health care, matter more than household income and local prices (measured independent of quality). Or it may be that results are poor because many studies are plagued by methodological problems.[7] Many studies of the determinants of health do not actually test directly the effects of truly exogenous variables such as prices (e.g., of food or health services, or of labor—i.e., wages), or they do so in an estimation that also includes improperly specified endogenous variables. Endogenous variables are those that already reflect choices made by the household; if the estimation does not take into account their endogeneity (either by excluding them and estimating a reduced-form equation, or by using simultaneous estimation techniques to purge them of endogeneity), then results can be misleading. For example, if estimates do not take into account the likelihood that sick mothers or children are least able to breast-feed, the apparent positive effects of breast-feeding on children's good health will be overstated. If estimates fail to take into account that very sick children are those most likely to be taken to the health clinic, the positive impact of clinic visits in reducing child mortality will be understated. Worse still, if researchers fail to take into account the possibility that governments are giving priority to placing health services where sickness and mortality are high, the possible positive effects of services on mortality may be understated.[8] Epidemiological studies of specific diseases without adequate control groups are likely to suffer from these types of estimation problems.[9]

In short, household-level analyses have not been definitive on the effects of variables that represent policy interventions such as availability or price of health services. However, in these analyses there has been a constant process of advance in understanding, as conceptual and methodological problems have been successively encountered, grappled with, and overcome. Conceptual advances have led to changes in data collection efforts, which have in turn simplified methodological problems. An example is the growing emphasis in data collection efforts on incorporation of community-level variables that represent well exogenous "prices" to the household, including, most recently, information on actual cash prices of alternative health services.[10]

At the national level, high per capita income is not in itself critical to better health. Though some minimal level of income is almost surely a prerequisite to maintaining good health, that level is fairly low. Above the level, other factors matter as much if not more. Much improvement in health has occurred as a result of development in the broadest sense, not because of improvements in personal health services. Cross-national studies suggest that in the first two or three decades of the postwar period, improvements in the technology of disease control, in transportation and communication, and in food distribution during emergencies[11] were important contributors to better health. Many of these factors required no change in health systems in developing countries to bring about lower mortality, and little or no change in individual attitudes or behavior. In this sense, development in the broadest sense has contributed, and should continue to contribute, to better health.

On the other hand, the relative power of factors that do not rely on changes in individual behavior on simple one-time acts (such as having children vaccinated) to contribute to ever-lower mortality may be declining. It is natural that diminishing returns to simple widespread interventions such as antimalarial spraying would set in wherever mortality is relatively low (e.g., where the infant mortality rate is below 100 per thousand births).[12] This would imply that in the future the effects of development on health are likely to be observed more and more through changes in individual behavior and changes in such factors as education, access to information, and—possibly—greater access to critical (mostly preventive) health care services that have the potential to affect individual health behavior.

Education, especially of mothers, is a critical determinant of children's health.[13] In some settings, it probably substitutes for better sanitation (Merrick 1985) and for greater availability of care and vice versa (Rosenzweig and Schultz 1982), possibly because availability of both care and education reduce the costs to mothers of getting and exploiting information on how to care for children.

Estimates using the Cebu, Philippines, study indicate that mother's education can result in reduced diarrhea by increasing food intake, increasing use of preventive health services, and improving personal hygiene practices (Cebu Study Team 1991). At the household level, use of health services does not seem to make any differences to mortality. This is paradoxical, given that countries successful in reducing mortality, such as China and Sri Lanka, have emphasized access to basic health services. Of course, health services may matter more for morbidity than for mortality; few household studies have examined morbidity. And at the household level, much use of services is in direct response to illness, whereas the key to low mortality and morbidity in successful countries has been emphasis not on curative services or even services per se but on preventive care through outreach. It is also worth noting that China, Sri Lanka, Cuba, and other successful countries have had extensive and effective food distribution systems and relatively well-educated populations.

In developing countries, use of health services does not appear to be particularly price-elastic, except for the poor. For the average consumer and within certain ranges, the price of health services has little effect on their use by consumers (see Akin, Guilkey, Griffin, and Popkin 1985; Akin, Birdsall, and de Ferranti 1987). But at the same time, and this is not surprising, prices do matter for the poor, for whom a higher price represents, other things being equal, a bigger chunk of income (Gertler, Dor, Locay, Sanderson, and van der Gaag 1988). On the one hand, insofar as use of health services does not matter for mortality, it may not seem important that prices discourage use of services by the poor. On the other hand, use of even simple curative services may have important welfare effects, if it relieves pain and anxiety. And existing studies may not sufficiently differentiate between the effects of use of different kinds of services; if high prices discourage use of particularly effective services (e.g., prenatal care), health costs (including mortality) may be higher than so far demonstrated.

Finally, poor nutrition makes good health unlikely, but poor health also exacerbates malnutrition by reducing nutrient absorption. It is possible that specific nutrient deficiencies as well as protein-calorie malnutrition have profound effects on health that are not easily addressed through health services.[14]

A final two-part conclusion does not come directly from the literature, but it can be inferred. It concerns public expenditures on health. First, these expenditures are only one input to improved health; many other factors (education, transportation, food prices and distribution, even food habits) matter and may matter more. Second, the effect of public expenditures on health is highly dependent on the allocation of those expenditures between cost-effective activities (basic health services, endemic disease control—largely but not exclusively preventive) and high-cost hospital services.

Potential for Breaking New Ground

Many questions critical for improving health policy and, thus, health in developing countries remain unanswered. Four potentially fruitful areas of new research are:

- Additional studies in more settings of several critical aspects of household behavior, for example, by what mechanisms mother's education makes a difference to child health (and whether there are quick substitutes for mother's education); and whether and how much the price of health care (and of private insurance) makes a difference to use of services of various kinds

- Analysis of the political economy of public expenditures on health—the determinants and composition of public spending on health, including the poor allocation of public resources between largely private goods, especially high-cost hospital care, and the largely public good activities that are more cost-effective in improving health, such as basic health services, disease control, nutritional and epidemiological surveillance

- Analysis of alternative financing mechanisms for health care, and alternative mechanisms for controlling costs

- New work on concepts, methods, and data needs for study of adult health, including not only adult mortality but also adult morbidity

Work on the cost-effectiveness of alternative health-enhancing inputs (e.g., doctors versus nurses, vaccines versus drugs) is critical for the design of health programs and could certainly constitute another category. Such work is an input (in effect a tool) for work in other categories, as will become evident in our subsequent discussion.

Household level studies. Studies of the effects of various measures of development on health at the cross-national level can generate hypotheses but cannot be conclusive, since they cannot capture variations in the endowments and the price environment of individuals and households, which ultimately are what matter. The potential for breaking new ground is thus at the household level, where, despite a large body of literature using increasingly sophisticated methodology,[15] the potential for policy-relevant results has been limited until recently by data problems.

For example, as we have noted, in studies to date the effects of prices (of food, health services, etc.) on health have appeared to be surprisingly small. But only recently have household surveys begun to combine information at the household level on income and expenditures for other services as well as health, with the necessary information at the community level on quantity, quality and user prices of health care, related services, food, transportation, and so forth. Information on other consumption and the prices of other services is necessary because even if households do not reduce use of health services in the face of higher prices for health care, they may be reducing consumption of other goods or services that affect health, such as food or education, or they may be reallocating their spending in other ways that imply large reductions in both family welfare and social welfare. Detailed information on the range of health services is necessary because consumers may switch among suppliers (and have high price elasticities across suppliers, though a low elasticity for health services overall).

For adequate study of the mechanisms by which mother's education affects child health, conventional quantitative household survey data probably need to be combined with information on attitudes, day-to-day behavior, and the intrafamilial bargaining process. Specific controlled experiments of effects of interventions across households with different educational profiles could also have high payoff in generating new hypotheses. The potential for new work on the effects of education on health has been outlined recently by Caldwell (1989).

The political economy of public spending on health. Research in this area could contribute to greatly improved public debate on the appropriate role of government in health. There are at least four critical areas of work. One, alternative models of health finance and provision, is set out as a separate category below. A second is empirical and conceptual work on the actual and appropriate roles of the public versus the private (nonprofit and for-profit) sectors in financing and provision of care, and in provision of information, regulation, and other nonservice aspects of health care. Empirical work should include analyses of the relative efficiency of the public and private sectors in health in developing countries; these are rare, if only for lack of good data on costs.[16]

A third area of work is development of a theory of "good government," one that would explain variations across countries in the efficiency and equity of public expenditures for health (and other programs). Technical analyses by the World Bank and others tend to indicate that in health, most countries face no real tradeoff between equity and efficiency; for example, a reallocation of spending from high-cost hospital care to basic services in rural areas would both improve aggregate health indicators and better serve the poor.[17] Birdsall and James (1990) note that many governments persist in patterns of spending for health and other social programs despite this lack of tradeoff, apparently because the current pattern better serves those with political power and influence. They also note that alterations in that apparent equilibrium have and do occur; for example, in response to exogenous shocks to the political system or new information from outside the system. Recent analyses in a few countries of the effects of macroeconomic adjustment (or lack of adjustment) on health outcomes provide a start in this area, since they involve study of changes in expenditure patterns as a function of a kind of exogenous shock to the system (in this case changes in the macroeconomic environment.)[18]

Finally, work on the optimal ratio between curative and preventive interventions, and the optimal allocation of responsibility for coverage of each between the public purse (e.g., funded by general revenues or nationwide insurance mechanisms) and the private purse, would provide a benchmark for normative judgments about overall patterns of public spending on health. In spite of the near-consensus that preventive care receives inadequate public spending (and inadequate private spending as well), it is clear that some curative care must be provided (well beyond that portion of curative care that has high externalities, such as care of tubercular patients), and even financed publicly. For example, in a practical sense it may be difficult to convince consumers to use preventive care if needed referrals to adequate curative care are not possible; and of course there are economies of scope in the combined provision of preventive and curative care.[19] In addition, it can be argued that all individuals benefit from the "option value" of availability of curative care, whether they ever actually use it or not. In the end, though, in many settings it is possible to say that too much is spent on high-cost hospital care and too little on largely preventive basic care. The existing literature is virtually silent on the appropriate balance and criteria for determining that balance.

Some insight on this issue is likely to come from the small but growing body of literature on the cost-effectiveness of health interventions in industrialized countries. Insights from these include the following points (Barnum and Kutzin 1990; Jamison and Mosley 1992);

- Most primary prevention activities (such as health promotion campaigns against smoking and alcohol abuse and for exercise and use of motorcycle helmets) are "good buys".
- Some secondary prevention activities (such as cervical cancer screening and physical screening for breast cancer) are good buys; but many common secondary prevention activities (such as hypertension screening programs) are not cost-effective.
- Many treatment procedures are not cost-effective, but some (including pacemaker implantation, hip replacements, and treating of breast and cervical cancer, and even some coronary bypass surgery) are cost-effective.

The limitations of this literature are still very great. Research has primarily been devoted to assessing the cost-effectiveness of medical procedures in industrialized countries. It is fraught with fundamental methodological and empirical problems. Additional work in this area is vital, both to clarify the outstanding questions and, prior to this, to force policymakers to ask the right questions and think correctly.

Finally, in the area of the political economy of health spending, there is scope for much international comparative analysis. However, a preliminary step is thorough analysis at the national level of public investment and expenditure trends and their determinants in a range of developing countries. This kind of work is increasingly being undertaken at the World Bank, as health and other social sectors are now more frequently covered in general country reviews. These studies, to the extent they share a common conceptual framework, can eventually provide a basis for comparative work.

The rationale for work on the political economy of public spending on health, the simple analytics that might underline such work, and some of the central issues are outlined further in Birdsall (1989) and Birdsall (1992).[20]

Alternative financing and cost control mechanisms. This category is actually a large but important subset of the previous category. Systematic studies of alternative approaches to the financing (and provision) of health care in developed countries (e.g., Canada, Britain, and the United States), with a focus on their potential lessons for developing countries, are still rare. Yet a critical concern for developing countries is how to have reasonable health care without duplicating the experience of many developed countries with their large and rapidly rising share of resources in gross domestic product (GDP) devoted to health. There has been virtually no research on alternative approaches to health insurance (and to social insurance more generally) and its effects on health outcomes in developing countries. Systematic comparative studies and controlled experiments in developing countries (such as the Rand insurance study in California in the 1970s)[21] would have high payoff.

Even where health systems are highly decentralized and rely heavily on the private sector, the need to implement some forms of cost control seems reasonable. Alternative cost control mechanisms include (on the demand side) use of fees and insurance copayments and deductibles, and (on the supply side) rationing of access to medical school, to expensive technologies, and to drugs; centralized controls on the prices and number of procedures, including diagnostic-related group pricing; and use of preferred providers and other related mechanisms by those who are financing health, such as employers or insurance systems. Though these mechanisms are increasingly employed in developing countries, especially in Latin America,[22] and greater recourse to them is widely discussed, little empirical work has been done on their effects in reducing costs relative to any effects on health outcomes in developing countries.

Adult health. Additional work on the three topics just mentioned will be dependent on improvement in data and methodology for study of adult health, including adult mortality but especially adult morbidity. Table 9.1 provides a rough summary of this author's knowledge of the extent of the literature relating health and development; it compares work on determinants and development; it compares work on determinants and consequences of child (including infant) and adult mortality and morbidity.

Under determinants (our concentration in this section), I know of little work in developing countries on adult mortality and virtually no work on adult morbidity.[23] This is surprising since most societies allocate resources in a manner that apparently places a higher priority on reducing adult deaths and adult morbidity than reducing infant mortality; in many developed countries, the bulk of health spending is concentrated on the very old. What lies behind what economists would call a revealed preference for better adult health over reductions in infant and child mortality?[24] In the developed countries there is growing attention to economic analysis of problems of medical ethics, especially on the question of optimal spending on heroic measures to extend the lives of the elderly. Analytic work on these issues may be even more important in the developing countries, where resources are scarcer, government's role in centralized decisions regarding resource use is often greater, and the biases that arise from an unequal distribution of income may exacerbate distortions in use of health resources. One example of such work would be analysis of household behavior regarding health that examines the demand for health in the broadest sense, including the demand for

Table 9.1

Studies on Health and Development in Developing Countries

	Determinants	Consequences	Data Availability and Quality
Infant and child mortality	Extensive	Nil	Good
	Examples: Rosenzweig and Schultz (1982); Thomas, Strauss, and Henriques (1990)		
Infant and child morbidity	Extensive	Limited	Good
	Examples: Cebu Study Team (1991); Wolfe and Behrman (1987)	*Examples*: Moock and Leslie (1986); Salkever (1982)''	
Adult mortality	Limited	Nil	Poor
Adult morbidity	Limited	Limited	Poor
	(World Bank, 1989)	*Examples*: Strauss (1986); Deolalikar (1988)	

'' This study uses data from the United States.

relief of pain and suffering associated with adult noncommunicable diseases and adult disability.

Similarly, analysis of the political economy of health spending, particularly of the political impetus behind rising costs, will not be fruitful without new work on the costs and determinants (and consequences) of adult morbidity. The epidemiological transition is already upon us in many countries of the developing world, bringing relatively higher incidence of "adult" chronic diseases alongside the continuing high incidence of childhood infectious diseases. Data on the incidence and distribution (across age and socioeconomic groups) of adult morbidity, including injuries and disability, are critical to analysis of the likely effects of income growth and the aging of populations on the demand and overall costs of health care in developing countries, and to the design of prevention and health promotion programs. A striking example is available from Briscoe's analysis of Brazilian data (World Bank 1989). He shows that if various kinds of injuries are combined, including auto crashes, homicide, and suicide, the category of injuries accounts for more potential years of life lost for those aged 1 to 65 years than any other category (such as cancers, infectious and parasitic diseases, cardiovascular disease). Yet there is virtually no organized research on the topic of injuries in developing countries.[25]

Eventual Difference Research Might Make

Research on household demand for health and on health behavior would obviously contribute to better design of public health and nutrition programs, for example, by improving understanding of how education improves health and whether and how public information and services can substitute in the short run for education. It could lead to more sustainable financing of health care, through greater understanding of whether and how to implement user charges and how to rely on private sector programs without prejudicing public health goals or restricting access of the poor to health services. Health planners have naturally tended to focus on problems of the health system—supply-side problems—as the critical constraint to improving health. A great advantage of household studies is their emphasis on the demand side, on beneficiaries as consumers, and on behavior, including health-seeking behavior.

Research on the political economy of public expenditures on health would broaden the nature of health policy discussion in the international public health community beyond the (important and relatively well-understood) area of primary health care, and it could contribute to improvements in the public management (including regulation, quality control, and monitoring of private provision of health care) and financing of health care. Research in this area would also help to clarify the role of the nonmedical community and nonmedical public agencies in health care (e.g., highway safety, occupational health, regulation of food and drugs, public information regarding the health effects of diet, smoking, alcohol, drug abuse, and exercise).

Research on financing and cost control issues in developed countries is flourishing; some of the emerging lessons are relevant for developed countries. But differences in income, in the organization of health systems, and in the adequacy of capital and insurance markets mean such work must also be carried out in developing countries if they are to fully benefit. Such research would contribute to more sustainable programs and to greater realism about tradeoffs in spending within health systems.

Research on adult health would open up entire new frontiers; it could link the work on household behavior with work on the political economy of health spending, since it is adults who make the decisions regarding the allocation of household resources to health and who influence allocation of public resources across and within sectors. Research on adult health is critical to setting priorities within the health system and to the design of health programs to prevent and control noncommunicable disease and injuries. Finally, research on the determinants of adult health would generate a set of concepts and data that are essential for analysis of the consequences of the health of populations for the development of their countries.

EFFECTS OF HEALTH ON DEVELOPMENT

State of the Art

Economists have long theorized about the possible effects of poor health on labor productivity and, thus, income growth in developing economies. The efficiency wage hypothesis (Leibenstein 1957; Stiglitz 1976), for example, posits that employers in developing countries may pay wages above market rates because below a certain wage employees will be less productive due to poor health or nutrition. More recently, economists working on the modeling of economic growth have built upon possible externalities in human resources (with more emphasis on education and knowledge than on health, but not excluding health) (Azariadis and Drazen 1990).[26]

It seems likely that some level of good health in a population may generate positive externalities that cannot be captured by particular (healthy) individuals but that are shared by society as a whole in the form of more rapid economic growth. However, compared to the extensive literature on the determinants of health (and thus on the effects of various indicators of development on health), there is much less work on the effects of health on development—or on what might be called the consequences of health for development (see Table 9.1).

A number of reviews in the 1980s (Gwatkin 1983; Andreano and Helminiak 1988; Strauss 1985) concluded that the possible link between better health and greater productivity and income had not been established, either because research results of most studies were inconclusive or because the research methods used were flawed. There are good reasons for this lack of success.

First, studies that concentrate on the effects of individual health on simple output measures of labor productivity (e.g., the effects of anemia on labor productivity of sugarcane workers) might well be missing the much larger potential effect that better health would have through contributing to entrepreneurship, willingness to invest (including in education, job search, and so on), and creativity in general; these effects would be extraordinarily difficult to capture empirically. Second, as noted by Over, Ellis, Huber, and Solon (1989) in a recent thoughtful summary of work on the consequences of health for development, negative consequences of poor health may be difficult to document empirically because households and entire communities adopt coping mechanisms when illness strikes.[27] Coping may reduce the costs of poor health, but it may also itself entail costs. These costs may not be directly reflected in lost family income or reduced productivity. Costs may instead be reflected in reduced health of other family members, reduced consumption or foregone investment, reduced leisure of other family members, or even breakup of families. But costs such as these, especially costs imposed on other family members, have not generally been studied and are difficult to study without specially designed data.[28]

Despite these problems, there has been some success in establishing that better health contributes to higher productivity at the individual level. The increasing availability of data sets that include information on time use of household members, as well as income and own-production and measures of health, has permitted more definitive work on the issue. In their recent review, Behrman and Deolalikar (1988) put particular weight on recent studies by Strauss (1986) using data from Sierra Leone and Deolalikar (1988) using data from South India. These two authors report positive effects of "effective family labor" (itself a function of family labor hours and measures of food availability or anthropometry) on agricultural productivity. These studies are convincing because the authors take into account the likelihood that worker health status is itself an endogenous result of prior individual choices—and they still find separate effects of health status on labor productivity. Other recent studies by Moock and Leslie (1986) and Jamison (1986) suggest that nutritional status of children (in particular, height-for-age, a cumulative measure of nutritional status over time) affects school performance,[29] adding to the evidence that in general better health does speed development.

Better documentation of any effects of health status on productivity and income gains could, obviously, increase the interest of policymakers concerned with economic growth, in health. It is, however, only a first step. Ideally it should be possible to compare the benefits of investments in health (as a first step at least in terms of private income gains) to the costs of the investments that generated the additional income gains; such cost-benefit analysis would permit comparison of the rates of return to investments in health with rates of return to alternative investments (in, say, physical infrastructure, other social programs, and so on). In contrast to the large body of literature on the economic rates of return (private and social) to investment in education (based on increments in lifetime expected income as they are related to increments in education at the aggregate and individual level),[30] work on the private and social returns to investments in health is sparse indeed (but see Table 9.1 for a few studies of economic consequences of investments in health).

Potential for Breaking New Ground

Three fruitful approaches to new work on the consequences of health for development can be distinguished.

Productivity effects at the individual level. The first, on the labor and school productivity effects of health status at the household level (and indirectly on the private rate of return to investments in health), is typified by the work of Strauss, Deolalikar, and Jamison. This type of work is still in its infancy, and there is great potential for improved understanding if more of it is done.

Social cost-benefit analysis of health investments. The second approach is a cost-benefit analysis of health investments taking into account social as well as private costs and benefits.[31] Cost-benefit analysis of health investments is rare. Long-standing tradition in the health community that a value cannot and should not be put upon life has combined with daunting conceptual problems and poor data on costs to prevent the emergence of any strong research tradition of cost-benefit analysis of health investments, even in developed countries.

On the benefits side, the problem is valuation of health benefits in a manner that allows comparison of health to other benefits, for example, in monetary terms.[32] Alternative measures include use of the "human capital approach" which values additional days (or years) of healthy life in terms of the economic productivity of the individual's labor, and the "willingness-to-pay approach" which values health in terms of what people would pay to attain or keep it. Both present difficulties.

The human capital approach, for example, requires judgments on an appropriate rate for discounting future potential income and on whether and how to apply productivity weights. (Should an additional day of healthy life be valued identically for a baby and a productive adult? Should the life of someone who earns a low wage be valued less than that of someone who earns a high wage? It then requires further judgments on the weights to apply to different illnesses and to death, in order to distinguish among healthy days of life that would otherwise have been lost to death and to various degrees of morbidity and disability.[33]

The willingness-to-pay approach is likely to be distorted by income differences across households. For the same set of preferences, richer households are likely to have higher willingness to pay than poorer households.

In the end, it is difficult to place a value on a human life. Even if it were simple to do so, it would still be difficult to place a value on the social gains associated with general improvements in health in terms of creativity, entrepreneurial capacity, and other X-efficiency type measures (Leibenstein 1957), or on the avoidance of the costs to the families and communities of those individuals who suffer poor health.

On the cost side, researchers face great difficulties in obtaining good data, particularly in many developing countries where information systems are weak and public provision of much care through centralized systems lacking budget accountability has destroyed incentives to measure costs. The best work on costs has been done in connection with efforts to analyze the cost-effectiveness (i.e., the least costly way of achieving a certain goal) of different programs that fall under the rubric of primary health care.[34] Data on hospital costs and on costs of overall systems are even rarer.[35]

The potential for breaking new ground in cost-benefit analysis is huge in the long run but poor in the short run. In the current environment, academic researchers doing applied research inevitably are drawn to areas of work where (1) a research tradition has already developed (the paradigm is set); (2) methodological issues are relatively well drawn (though breakthroughs may be needed, the need itself is implicitly recognized); and (3) data are already available or the mechanisms for collecting data are well known. None of these factors obtains today.

Consequences of poor health for households and communities. The third approach is greater attention to the consequences of poor health for households and communities. This might be considered a sensible partial approach, concentrating on individual and community costs, to the larger challenge of cost-benefit analysis. Though little such work has been completed, World Bank staff are currently exploring the possibility of undertaking research along these lines, concentrating on the consequences of adult ill health. The feasibility of more general work on adult health issues (including measurement of adult mortality and study of the determinants of adult health) is also being explored. Any work on adult health would be likely to increase our understanding of the consequences of poor health for the development process.[36]

Eventual Difference Research Might Make

Research on the consequences of health for economic development could affect both the amount of public resources devoted to health and the allocation of such resources. In a world of scarce resources, there will inevitably be competing claims for resources for development programs, all of which are worthy in terms of delivering specific increments of improved welfare (e.g., an additional day of healthy life, an increment of ability to read and write, an increment of security in old age). If the short-term welfare benefits of two or more competing claims on society's resources are exactly equivalent, then the "productivity" of alternative investments (i.e., the effects on income-generating capacity) is and should be a decisive factor in choice of investments, since the additional income accruing to individuals as a result of the productivity factor is an input to long-term welfare.[37] There is little question that the literature on returns to education has influenced both the volume and the allocation of educational investments. This is most obviously the case among donors, who have consistently supported educational investments in developing countries and, in the last decade, have emphasized support to primary education because of its high social returns compared to secondary and higher education.[38] The health sector could similarly benefit.

Thus, the subject of the effects of health on development is one where good research would probably make a difference (by increasing the volume and improving the allocation of resources for health investments) but where the field is at least two decades behind the state of the art in education. The difficulties—in terms of concepts, data, and methods— are greatest in the area of economic and social consequences of adult ill health, both for the affected individual and his or her community; yet work on this issue is critical to cost-benefit analysis of health investments. Because so little has been done, the short-run returns to a major push in this area would be small and the risks of a long period of difficulty in reaching straightforward, widely accepted results are great. However, there are risks as well in failing to begin.

CONCLUSIONS

Research on the determinants of health at the household level could contribute to better design of public programs meant to improve health. This is particularly the case insofar as much future improvement in health in developing countries will rely on changes in behavior at the individual and household level. Research on the demand for health care (including the price elasticity of demand for health services), and on the effects of health service utilization on health itself, could improve pricing policies of governments and could contribute to design of mechanisms to control costs on the supply side as well. Work on the determinants of adult (as opposed to infant and child) health should be a high priority (adult morbidity as well as mortality), especially given the epidemiological and demographic transitions going on in virtually all developing countries. Better understanding of the political economy of health, especially of alternative financing and cost control mechanisms, combined with work on the determinants of adult health, will be critical to public policy to deal with the rising costs of health care, appropriate design and financing of health insurance, and the increasing need to emphasize prevention and control of adult chronic and degenerative disease.

More systematic analysis of the social returns to investments in health in developing countries may turn out to be absolutely necessary to support continuing increases in ever more costly health care. On the one hand, it is difficult to do cost-benefit analysis of health investments, in part because of the difficulty of valuing human life and of valuing a healthy and pain-free life as compared to a sick and painful one. And good health is a legitimate end in itself, central to individual welfare. On the other hand, other approaches are possible, including analysis of the effects of health status on individual productivity (at work and in school) and of the social and economic costs of poor health for families and communities. Efforts to measure the returns to investments in good health are critical in a world of scarcity, where the benefits of many worthwhile investments must be compared. Moreover, such efforts are likely to change not only our sense of how much to invest in health, but how to allocate such investments.

NOTES

1. Barlow (1979) reviewed the literature on health and development more than 10 years ago. His review is more thorough in covering the links among health, fertility, income, and nutrition, all of which he treats as endogenous variables in a general model of health and development.

2. A reader might ask: Why choose an objective of improved health rather than a broader overall development objective? A reasonable objective of economic development is to maximize the discounted sum of (current and future) individuals' "welfare." Health is widely acknowledged to be a critical input to individual welfare and thus is an objective in itself. In fact, several measures of health (life expectancy at birth and the infant mortality rate) are also widely viewed in the development literature as being among the single best proxy measures for overall development (where development generally refers to material, not necessarily political, welfare). Of course, making health an objective in itself does not provide guidance on its value relative to other components of welfare or of development; to do so would go far beyond the more modest objectives of this chapter.

3. Income probably has diminishing effects at high levels; additional income probably matters more to health for poorer individuals and poorer nations. See Musgrove and Heysen (1986) for a good illustration.

4. Of course, the other side of this coin (good health despite being poor) is why these societies, especially noncommunist Sri Lanka, have so often received relatively low economic returns on their large investments in human capital. Later in this chapter we will discuss the effects of health on development.

5. Thomas, Strauss, and Henriques (1990) find that the predicted logarithm of per capita expenditures, a proxy for income, does enhance child survival (when controlling for other factors including parents' education). They use a large data set from Brazil, where the range in income is probably greater than in many household data sets.

6. Even the importance of mother's education has been questioned. See Wolfe and Behrman (1987).

7. Behrman and Deolalikar (1988) point out the methodological implications of an important distinction between two categories of analysis. The first includes analyses of either the household demand for health outcomes (e.g., infant mortality) or the household demand for health goods (e.g., the utilization of health services or the purchase of inputs to health such as drugs). In these cases, the dependent variable should be estimated as a reduced form, that is, solely as a function of variables exogenous to the household, such as wages, the price of food, and the price of health care. An example of such an analysis of health outcomes is that of Rosenzweig and Schultz (1982), in which child mortality in Colombia is estimated as a function of such variables as mother's education and age and community-level food prices and availability of services. Rosenzweig and Schultz find that in that setting, greater availability of services does contribute to lower child mortality, especially for urban households in which mother's education is low (so that services may substitute for low maternal education). See also Strauss (1990) and Barrera (1990). An example of an analysis of the utilization of services can be found in Akin, Guilkey, Griffin, and Popkin (1985), in which the household's use of and choice of type of medical service are analyzed as a function of household variables and the case and time costs of using alternative services.

The second category of analysis is estimation of a health production function. For example, mortality or anthropometric indicators are estimated as a function or output of a set of input variables. Many of these variables, such as utilization of health care, breast-feeding, and consumption of food (and thus nutrient intake), are endogenous (i.e., are the result of choices made by household members) and should be treated as such; others, such as prices, wages, and parental endowment (e.g., education and height), are exogenous. (For an example, see Pitt and Rosenzweig 1985).

8. Rosenzweig and Wolpin (1986) provide some impressive evidence on the endogenous location of public health services. This could be a problem with the findings of Rosenzweig and Schultz (1982), reported in the preceding note.

9. Noneconomists have also developed models that take into account endogeneity (Mosley and Chen 1984; Briscoe, Akin, and Guilkey 1990).

10. Such community-level data have been collected in a few settings, most notably for health in the case of the Cebu (Philippines) study undertaken by researchers at the University of North Carolina, and in surveys sponsored by the World Bank as part of its Living Standards Measurement Study program. In the Cebu study, community-level data have been collected on prices, services availability, and quality of health care, as well as access to transportation. For examples of use of such data, see Gertler and van der Gaag (1988), Akin, Guilkey, Griffin, and Popkin (1985), and Cebu Study Team (1991).

Unfortunately, even these prices may not be immune from endogeneity. Rosenzweig and Wolpin (1989) explore the possibility of migration in response to community prices, which—if it occurs—raises questions about the exogeneity of such "prices."

11. These factors, not included in the analyses, are assumed to explain the "unexpected" improvements in life expectancy reported by Preston (1980) and by Wheeler (1980).

12. For additional discussion of this point, see Birdsall (1980; 1989)

13. Wolfe and Behrman (1987) argue that much of what appears to be education may simply reflect family background characteristics that are not observed. Their findings have not been duplicated, and they may result from the fact that educated siblings contribute during childhood to cognitive development of siblings who ultimately receive less formal education; or from a narrow range of differences in education across siblings. Moreover, using the same data set, the authors recently reported that differences in education across adult sibling mothers are reflected in changes in their own health (Behrman and Wolfe 1989).

14. For example, there is growing evidence that vitamin A deficiency increases susceptibility to mortality as a result of measles. See World Health Organization (1988).

15. It is of some concern that this line of research, increasingly sophisticated in methodology, is carried out by a relatively small group of economists, most of whom are located in a limited number of centers (at Yale, Pennsylvania, North Carolina, Minnesota). The requirements in terms of training and know-how for success in this area of research are relatively stringent, and low-skilled workers in this vineyard tend to produce work that because of methodological problems is not useful. The Cebu group based at North Carolina (see Note 10) have begun to bridge this gap by publishing their results in epidemiology journals and by pointing out the links between the approach economists have taken and approaches such as that taken by Mosley and Chen (1984); see Cebu Study Team (1991).

16. For example, in Brazil a hospitalization in a public hospital costs the social security agency 200 percent more than a hospitalization in a private hospital. The key question is whether this difference is accounted for by the possibility that public hospitals treat more difficult cases. Differences in pathology alone appear to be of limited importance, but it does appear that public hospitals (where mortality rates are about 70 percent higher) do see more severely ill patients (World Bank 1989). For further discussion of the private sector in health, see Griffin (1989).

Much more on the relative efficiency of the private and public sectors has been done in the education area. See, for example, James (1988a, 1988b) and Jimenez, Lockheed, and Paqueo (1991).

17. See, for example, Psacharopoulos, Tan, and Jimenez (1986) on education spending and Akin, Birdsall, and de Ferranti (1987) on health spending.

18. Best known are the studies sponsored by UNICEF. Behrman (1988) and Pan American Health Organization (1989) conclude that the impact of the macroeconomic crisis on health care and health outcomes has not been great.

19. See Birdsall (1989b) for discussion of this point in more detail.

20. For a critique of the former, see Reich (1992).

21. See Manning, Newhouse, Keeler, Benjamin, Dun, Leibowitz, Marquis, and Zwanziger (1987).

22. See World Bank (1989) for a summary at the country level of use of these mechanisms, covering chiefly North and South America and Europe.

23. See World Bank (1989) for assessment of the data on adult health in Brazil, a developing country with more information than most.

24. I am grateful to William McGreevey for stating this problem in terms of revealed preference. He notes:

Research needs to help reformulate our use of indicators in such manner as to assure that the indicators adequately reflect revealed preference and not just an imposed value judgment implicit, for example, in a narrowly conceived program such as UNICEF GOBI strategy that only emphasizes the needs of one age segment of the population. (McGreevey, personal communication)

Revealed preference in most countries suggests heavy preference weights for adult health, even taking into account that the unit costs of dealing with adult morbidity are higher than unit costs of dealing with infant mortality. In the United States, a study by the Institute of Medicine attempted to elicit judgments from health professionals on the relative undesirability of death at different ages. The death of an adult (age 15 to 59) was judged by those interviewed as being 2.5 to 10 times more undesirable than the death of a child. The death of a person 60 years or older was judged to be 0.2 to 0.1 times more undesirable than the death of a child.

25. See Jamison and Mosley (1992, forthcoming) for an impressive effort to tackle health sector priorities by looking across disease and injury categories.

26. See also Lucas (1988) and Romer (1986).

27. For example, households that include sick members are more likely to receive private transfers from other households, as documented by Cox and Jimenez (1989).

28. Salkever (1982) estimated using U.S. data on families with handicapped children that the hidden costs included at least an estimated $1 billion (in 1975 dollars) of lost family income due to reduced maternal working hours. This appears to be one of the few such studies of the costs of foregone labor of parents of disabled children.

29. Behrman and Deolalikar (1988) note that these studies may be misleading if certain children are both healthier and do better in school, with no causal impact of the former on the latter.

30. For a recent review of the literature on the private and social rates of return to education, including in developing countries, see Psacharopoulos (1985). Behrman and Birdsall (1987) review a number of studies suggesting that the estimated private returns (though not necessarily social returns) reported by Psacharopoulos are probably biased upward, for a variety of reasons, but are still high relative to private rates of returns to many physical investments in developing countries. Haveman and Wolfe (1984) point out that social returns to education may be underestimated because they fail to take into account such likely positive externalities as the effects of education on improving health.

31. This would be distinct from the cost-effectiveness analysis discussed previously. Cost-effectiveness analysis compares the costs of alternative approaches

to achieving a specific health objective. Cost-benefit analysis compares the social benefits of investing in health versus nonhealth investments.

32. This is not necessary for comparing the benefits of alternative health investments, as in cost-effectiveness analysis. Only benefits in terms of improved health (e.g., additional days of healthy life) are then necessary.

33. See Barnum (1987) for application of weights to epidemiological data from Ghana.

34. See Abel-Smith (1989) for a discussion of cost-effectiveness. He cites work by Mills (1985).

35. But see Barnum and Kutzin (1990).

36. Regarding the World Bank's recent efforts, see Over, Ellis, Huber, and Solon (1989) and Feachem (1989). The World Bank has also recently completed two country studies of Brazil and China, each with a heavy concentration on issues of adult health (World Bank 1989; 1990).

37. Some would argue that additional income at some point would reduce health status, as more people smoke, as the risks of traffic injuries rise with more cars, and so forth. It is true that the effects of productivity gains on health status are not necessarily clear, since the effects of income on health are not clear. It is clear, however, that the effects of productivity gains on welfare (as opposed to health, which may be one argument of the welfare function) will be positive. If higher income allows people to choose to live shorter but happier lives (because they enjoy smoking or eating red meat), their welfare if not their health has improved.

38. The World Bank has consistently emphasized the high rates of return to education in its publications, including the *World Development Reports* of 1980, 1981, 1984; and in policy studies of financing education (1986) and of education issues in Africa (1988b).

REFERENCES

Abel-Smith, B. 1989. Health Economics in Developing Countries. *Journal of Tropical Medicine and Hygiene* 92:229–41.

Akin, J., N. Birdsall, and D. de Ferranti. 1987. *Financing Health in Developing Countries: An Agenda for Reform.* Washington, D.C.: World Bank.

Akin, J. S., D. Guilkey, C. Griffin, and B. Popkin. 1985. *The Demand for Primary Health Services in the Third World.* Totowa, New Jersey: Rowman and Allanheld Publishers.

Andreano, R., and T. Helminiak. 1988. Economics, Health and Tropical Diseases: A Review. In *Economics, Health and Tropical Diseases.* A. N. Herrin and P. L. Rosenfield, eds. Manila: University of Philippines, School of Economics.

Azariadis, C., and A. Drazen. 1990. Threshold Externalities in Economic Development. *Quarterly Journal of Economics* 105:501–26.

Barlow, R. 1979. Health and Economic Development: A Theoretical and Empirical Review. *Research in Human Capital and Development* 1:45–75.

Barnum, H. 1987. Evaluating Healthy Days of Life Gained from Health Projects. *Social Science and Medicine* 24:833–41.

Barnum, H., and J. Kutzin. 1990. *Patterns of Hospital Resource Use in Developing Countries*. PHN Technical Note. Washington, D.C.: World Bank.

Barrera, A. 1990. The Role of Maternal Schooling and Its Interaction with Public Health Programs in Child Health Production. *Journal of Development Economics* 32:69–91.

Behrman, J. R. 1988. Intrahousehold Allocation of Nutrients in Rural India: Are Boys Favored? Do Parents Exhibit Inequality Aversion? *Oxford Economic Papers* 40:32–54.

Behrman, J. R., and A. B. Deolalikar. 1988. Health and Nutrition. In *Handbook of Development Economics*. H. Chenery and T. N. Srinivasan, eds. Amsterdam: North Holland.

Behrman, J. R., and B. L. Wolfe. 1987. How Does Mother's Schooling Affect the Family's Health, Nutrition, Medical Care Usage, and Household Sanitation? *Journal of Econometrics* 36:185–204.

———. 1989. Does More Schooling Make Women Better Nourished and Healthier? Adult Sibling Random and Fixed Effects Estimates for Nicaragua. *Journal of Human Resources* 24:644–63.

Behrman, J. R., and N. Birdsall. 1987. Communication on Returns to Education: A Further Update and Implications. *Journal of Human Resources* 22:4:603–606.

Birdsall, N. 1980. Population Growth and Poverty in the Developing World. *Population Bulletin* 35:5. Washington, D.C.: Population Reference Bureau, Inc.

———. 1989. Thoughts on Good Health and Good Government. *Daedalus* 118:1:89–117.

———. 1992. Pragmatism, Robin Hood and Other Themes: Good Government and Social Well-Being in Developing Countries. In *Social Dimensions of Health Transitions: An International Perspective*. L. C. Chen, A. M. Kleinman, and N. C. Ware, eds. New York: Oxford University Press, in preparation. Also published in *Population and Development Review*.

Birdsall, N., and E. James. 1990. *Efficiency and Equity in Social Spending: How and Why Governments Misbehave* Population and Human Resources Working Paper Number 274. Washington, D.C.: World Bank.

Briscoe, J., J. Akin, and D. Guilkey. 1990. People Are Not Passive Acceptors of Threats to Health: Endogeneity and Its Consequences. *International Journal of Epidemiology* 19:1:147–53.

Caldwell, J. C. 1989. *Introductory Thoughts on Health Transition*. Paper prepared for the workshop on Cultural, Social, and Behavioral Determinants of Health: What Is the Evidence? Canberra, Australia.

Cebu Study Team. 1991. Underlying and Proximate Determinants of Child Health: The Cebu Longitudinal Health and Nutrition Study. *American Journal of Epidemiology* 133:2:185–201.

Cox, D., and E. Jimenez. 1989. *Private Transfers and Public Policy in Developing Countries: A Case Study for Peru*. PPR Working Paper No. 345. Washington, D.C.: World Bank.

Deolalikar, A. B. 1988. Do Health and Nutrition Influence Labor Productivity in Agriculture? Econometric Estimates for Rural South India. *Review of Economics and Statistics* 70:2:406–13.

Feachem, R. G. 1989. *The Health of Adults in the Developing World.* Draft paper. Washington, D.C.: World Bank.

Feachem, R. G., W. G. Graham, and I. M. Timaeus. 1989. Identifying Health Problems and Health Research Priorities in Developing Countries. *Journal of Tropical Medicine and Hygiene* 92:133–91.

Gertler, P., and J. van der Gaag. 1988. *Measuring the Willingness to Pay for Social Services in Developing Countries.* LSMS Working Paper No. 45. Washington, D.C.: World Bank.

Gertler, P., A. Dor, L. Locay, W. Sanderson, and J. van der Gaag. 1988. *Health Care Financing and the Demand for Medical Care.* LSMS Working Paper No. 37. Washington, D.C.: World Bank.

Griffin, C. 1989. *Strengthening Health Services in Developing Countries through the Private Sector.* Discussion Paper No. 4. Washington, D.C.: International Finance Corporation.

Gwatkin, D. R. 1983. *Does Better Health Produce Greater Wealth? A Review of the Evidence concerning Health, Nutrition, and Output.* Washington, D.C.: Overseas Development Council.

Haddad, L., and H. E. Boris. 1989. *The Impact of Nutritional Status on Agricultural Productivity: Wage Evidence from the Philippines.* Development Economics Research Centre Discussion Paper 97. Warwick: University of Warwick.

Halstead, S. B., J. A. Walsh, and K. S. Warren, Eds. 1985. *Good Health at Low Cost.* New York: Rockefeller Foundation.

Haveman, R. H., and B. L. Wolfe. 1984. Schooling and Economic Well-Being: The Role of Nonmarket Effects. *Journal of Human Resources* 19:377–407.

James, E. 1988a. *The Relationship between Public and Private Sectors in Higher Education.* Report prepared for the International Academy of Education.

———. 1988b. *Public and Private Higher Education in the Philippines.* Washington, D.C.: World Bank.

Jamison, D. T. 1986. Child Malnutrition and School Performance in China. *Journal of Developmental Economics* 20:299–310.

Jamison, D. T., and W. H. Mosley. 1992. *Evolving Health Sector Priorities in Developing Countries.* Washington, D.C.: World Bank, forthcoming.

Jimenez, E., M. Lockheed, and V. Paqueo. 1991. The Relative Efficiency of Private and Public Schools in Developing Countries. *World Bank Research Observer* 6:2:205–18.

Leibenstein, H. A. 1957. *Economic Backwardness and Economic Growth.* New York: Wiley.

Lucas, R. 1988. On the Mechanics of Economic Development. *Journal of Monetary Economics* 21:3–42.

Manning, W. G., J. P. Newhouse, E. Keeler, B. Benjamin, N. Dun, A. Leibowitz, M. Marquis, and J. Zwanziger. 1987. *Health Insurance and the Demand for Medical Care: Evidence from a Randomized Experiment.* Report No. R.3476-HHS. Santa Monica, Calif.: Rand Corporation.

Martorell, R., and G. Arroyave. 1984. *Malnutrition, Work Output, and Energy Need.* Paper presented at the International Union of Biological Sciences Symposium on Variation in Working Capacity in Tropical Populations. London, England.

Merrick, T. W. 1985. The Effect of Piped Water on Early Childhood Mortality in Urban Brazil, 1970–1976. *Demography* 22:1–24.

Mills, A. 1985. Survey and Examples of Economic Evaluation of Health Programmes in Developing Countries. *World Health Statistics Quarterly* 38:4:402–31.

Moock, P., and J. Leslie. 1986. Childhood Malnutrition and Schooling in the Terai Region of Nepal. *Journal of Development Economics* 20:33–52.

Mosley, W. H. 1992. Potential for Social Science Research to Inform and Influence the Delivery of Health Care in Less Developed Countries. In *Advancing Health in Developing Countries: The Role of Social Research*. L. C. Chen, A. M. Kleinman, and N. C. Ware, eds. Westport, Conn.: Auburn House.

Mosley, W. H., and L. C. Chen. 1984. An Analytic Framework for the Study of Child Survival in Developing Countries. *Population and Development Review* 10:25–48.

Musgrove, P., and S. Heysen. 1986. Interdepartmental Differences in Life Expectancy at Birth in Peru as It Relates to Income, Household Drinking Water, and Provision of Medical Consultations. *Bulletin of the Pan-American Health Organization* 20:1:31–44.

Over, M., R. Ellis, J. Huber, and O. Solon. 1989. The Consequences of Adult Ill Health. Draft prepared for the World Bank, December.

Pan American Health Organization. 1989. *Health and Development: Repercussion of the Economic Crisis*. Report No. CE103/7. Washington, D.C.: PAHO.

Pitt, M. M., and M. R. Rosenzweig. 1985. Health and Nutrient Consumption across and within Farm Households. *Review of Economics and Statistics* 67:212–23.

Preston, S. H. 1980. Causes and Consequences of Mortality Declines in Less Developed Countries during the Twentieth Century. In *Population and Economic Change in Developing Countries*. R. A. Easterlin, ed. Chicago: University of Chicago Press.

———. 1983. *Mortality and Development Revisited*. Philadelphia: University of Pennsylvania. Mimeo.

Psacharopoulos, G. 1985. Returns to Education: A Further International Update and Implications. *Journal of Human Resources* 20:584–604.

Psacharopoulos, G., J. P. Tan, and E. Jimenez. 1986. *Financing Education in Developing Countries*. Washington, D.C.: World Bank.

Rashad, H. 1989. Oral Rehydration Therapy and Its Effect on Child Mortality in Egypt. *Journal of Biosocial Science Supplement* 10:105–13.

Reich, M. 1992. The Political Economy of Health Transitions. In *Social Dimensions of Health Transitions: An International Perspective*. L. C. Chen, A. M. Kleinman, and N. C. Ware, eds. New York: Oxford University Press, in preparation.

Romer, P. M. 1986. Increasing Returns and Long-Run Growth. *Journal of Political Economy* 94:5:1002–1036.

Rosenzweig, M. R., and K. J. Wolpin. 1986. Evaluating the Effects of Optimally Distributed Public Programs. *American Economic Review* 76:470–87.

———. 1989. Migration Selectivity and the Effects of Public Programs. *Journal of Public Economics* 37:3:265–89.

Rosenzweig, M. R., and T. P. Schultz. 1982. Child Mortality and Fertility in Colombia: Individual and Community Effects. In *Health Policy and Education*, vol. 2. Amsterdam: Elsevier Scientific Publishing Co.

———. 1989. Market Opportunities, Genetic Endowments, and Intrafamily Resource Distribution: Child Survival in Rural India. *American Economic Review* 72:803–15.

Salkever, D. S. 1982. Children's Health Problems: Implications for Parental Labor Supply and Earnings. In *Economic Aspects of Health*. V. R. Fuchs, ed. Chicago: University of Chicago Press.

Schwartz, J. B., J. S. Akin, and B. M. Popkin. 1988. Price and Income Elasticities of Demand for Modern Health Care: The Case of Infant Deliveries in the Philippines. *World Bank Economic Review*, 2:1:49–76.

Stevens, C. M. 1977. Health and Economic Development: Longer-Run View. *Social Science and Medicine* 2:809–17.

Stiglitz, J. E. 1976. The Efficiency Wage Hypothesis, Surplus, Labour, and the Distribution of Income in LDCs. *Oxford Economic Papers, New Series* 28:185–207.

Strauss, J. 1985. *The Impact of Improved Nutrition in Labor Productivity and Human Resource Development: An Economic Perspective.* Economic Growth Center Discussion Paper No. 494. New Haven: Yale University.

———. 1986. Does Better Nutrition Raise Farm Productivity? *Journal of Political Economy* 94:297–320.

———. 1990. Households, Communities and Preschool Children's Nutrition Outcomes: Evidence from Rural Cote d'Ivoire. *Economic Development and Cultural Change* 38:231–61.

Thomas, D., J. Strauss, and M. Henriques. 1990. Child Survival, Height for Age and Household Characteristics in Brazil. *Journal of Development Economics* 33:197–234.

Wheeler, D. 1980. Basic Needs Fulfillment and Economic Growth: A Simultaneous Model. *Journal of Development Economics* 7:435–51.

Wolfe, B., and J. R. Behrman. 1987. Women's Schooling and Children's Health: Are the Effects Robust with Adult Sibling Control for the Women's Childhood Background? *Journal of Health Economics* 6:239–54.

World Bank. 1980. *World Development Report.* Washington, D.C.: World Bank.

———. 1981. *World Development Report.* Washington, D.C.: World Bank.

———. 1984. *World Development Report.* Washington, D.C.: World Bank.

———. 1986. *Financing Education in Developing Countries: An Exploration of Policy Options.* Washington, D.C.: World Bank.

———. 1988a. *Brazil—Public Spending on Social Programs: Issues and Options.* Report No. 7086-BR, vol. 1. Washington, D.C.: World Bank.

———. 1988b. *Education in Sub-Saharan Africa: Policies for Adjustment, Revitalization and Expansion.* Washington, D.C.: World Bank.

———. 1989. *Brazil—Adult Health in Brazil: Adjusting to New Challenges.* Report No. 7807-BR. Washington, D.C.: World Bank.

———. 1990. *China—Long-Term Issues and Options for the Health Sector.* Report No. 7965-CHA. Washington, D.C.: World Bank.

World Health Organization. 1988. *Expanded Progress on Immunization Programs for the Control of Vitamin A Deficiency: The Role of the EPI in New Initiatives for the 1990s.* WHO-EPI-GAG, Working Paper No. 11, Rev 1. Geneva, Switzerland: World Health Organization.

10

Potential for Social Science Research to Inform and Influence the Delivery of Health Care in Less Developed Countries

W. HENRY MOSLEY

INTRODUCTION

This discussion of the usefulness of social science research begins with a philosophical discourse on the expectations of the scientific endeavor in the social sciences. It is followed by an overview of the field of public health from an historical perspective in terms of contributions of the social sciences to its evolution. This leads into an analysis of what I feel are the challenges for the future that will determine whether social science research will, indeed, contribute fundamentally to the improvement of human health or only operate at the margins. All of this in a single chapter will require some broad generalizations to be made in discussing major subjects.

SCIENCE AND THE SOCIAL SCIENCES

In assessing the state of the art in social science research I want to take a somewhat philosophical view of the scientific endeavor by the disciplines encompassed under the rubric of social science. Much of my discussion will be guided by the recent work of Rubinstein and his colleagues (Rubinstein 1984; Rubinstein, Laughlin, and McManus 1984). At the risk of oversimplification, the social sciences could be dichotomized in terms of their view of what constitutes the "proper" study of human behavior. At one extreme are the disciplines in which the building blocks of knowledge are quantitative relationships, following the accepted tenets of the "scientific method." In large measure this group includes epidemiologists, sociologists, economists, and demographers. A premise of this approach to the investigation of human behavior is that the subjects of study are thought of as objects existing independently of the researcher. Good science in these fields requires adherence to certain techniques and forms of presentation including particular data-gathering methods and representative samples. For an explanation to be accepted as scientific it "must take a form such that the event to be explained is presented as a conclusion of an argument which essentially contains in it premises that specify some relevant initial conditions and some statistical generalizations or universal laws" (Rubinstein 1984: 166).

The other end of the spectrum is represented by the field of anthropology, which concentrates on understanding the "processes" in social life. In this approach it is accepted that there is a continual interaction between the researcher and subject. Even more significant is that the anthropologists is not restricted to a normatively mandated set of techniques but rather will draw on the "sensitive selective use of different ways of knowing which are appropriate for the questions being asked" (Rubinstein 1984: 167). The goal of anthropological research is to gain knowledge of the processes being investigated, that is, how behavioral outcomes occur.

This distinction between what constitutes scientific inquiry is important. The "positivist" view defines the legitimate domains of scientific inquiry as those limited to characteristics of populations that are subject to "objective" measurement by standardized techniques. Scientific knowledge means prediction. However, this approach, severely restricts the breadth and depth of information that may be gathered. The "pragmatist" approach to science and knowledge recognizes not only that researchers are not neutral and objective but that there are, in fact, processes in human social life that cannot be grasped by traditional quantitative techniques such as symbolism, intentionality, and consciousness. In this view, scientific explanation becomes an ongoing process of developing a deeper understanding of human behavior.

The objective of highlighting these distinctions is not to give one approach supremacy over the other; rather, it is to recognize both as necessary to the task of the social sciences. Impressive technological innovations and much of our understanding of the biosocial mechanisms of disease processes and human reproduction have come from the scientific approach based on positivist principles. We are coming to appreciate, however, that our base of knowledge about human behavior is severely limited by restricting ourselves to this approach and that there is a need for the pragmatist approach of developing new ways of knowing and understanding how the objectively measurable outcomes occur in human populations. Three examples of recent research illustrate the range of insights that can be gained by the most rigorous quantitative approaches, by highly subjective observations, and by a combination of the two.

Research by the Cebu Study Team

The Cebu Study Team (1991) brings together scientists with expertise in demography, economics, environmental sciences, epidemiology, nutrition, pediatrics, and statistics in a prospective follow-up of over 3,000 Filipino women through pregnancy and the first two years of their infants' lives. The objective of this research is to develop a coherent behavioral and biomedical model that defines, first, how the underlying individual, family, and community variables affect health- and non-health-related behaviors, and second, how the underlying and intermediate socioeconomic, behavioral, and biomedical variables affect the growth, morbidity, and mortality of a child. Critical attention has been given to the identification and objective measurement of a wide range of underlying, intermediate, and outcome variables, and to the specification of the structural equations that are used in the analyses. Sophisticated analytical techniques are used to control for such factors as "unobserved heterogeneity," lagged effects, selection biases, and sample selectivity in order to obtain statistically unbiased estimates of the relationships among the variables. This approach provides quantitative estimates of the effects of a one-year increase in maternal education on "intermediate behavioral variables" related to breast-feeding and dietary supplementation, health service use, and personal hygienic behaviors and, through these, to diarrhea incidence.

The integration of these disciplinary sciences clearly provides a comprehensive insight into the quantitative interrelationships among a multiplicity of factors that are related to health. But it should be noted that the strengths of this approach are also its weaknesses: Only variables that are predefined and objectively measurable are included, and all relationships must be specified a priori. This, of course, is the correct procedure for hypotheses testing, but it precludes discovery of new knowledge and generally leaves unanswered the deeper questions of how the relationships between the underlying and proximate variables come about, for example, how does one year of schooling actually influence breast-feeding, or does it at all?

Research by Bledsoe

The report by Bledsoe (1989), "Foster Children and the Phenomenon of Scrounging," provides a contrasting illustration of the importance in scientific inquiry of being willing to develop innovative methods of research that are sensitive to the particular problem under study. Becoming aware that stealing was an important strategy for child survival, Bledsoe recognized that "needed were some occasionally unconventional methods to elicit sensitive information about the child culture of stealing on the gamble that it could yield rich insight" (Bledsoe 1989: 2). Among the techniques utilized were "inadvertent and highly serendipitous" use of participant observation, open-ended interviewing of adults and children, meal simulations, and encouraging children to maintain diaries.

In discussing the analytical implications of her research strategy, Bledsoe refers to a revolutionary shift in social-cultural theory from a mechanistic and static explanation of the cultural determinants of behavior to the pursuit of "processual questions." Specifically, she states:

We also need to talk less about cultural "traditions" or "customs" and more about the dynamics of economics, power and stratification . . . Our explanations also need to incorporate people's strategic attempts to influence each other's felt obligations and to step outside the formal bounds of households. Attempting to locate explanations of messy ambiguous behavior in what we might call the "structure in the strategies"—how people actually use or manipulate cultural norms and categories to shape health or nutritional outcomes—tends to stretch the patience of analysts who strive for numerical and social clarity. (Bledsoe 1989: 13)

Research by Schuler

In the study of "Barriers to Effective Family Planning in Nepal" by a group of anthropologists and physicians, Schuler, McIntosh, Goldstein, and Pande (1985) used "simulated" clients to investigate why family planning services are underused. The goal was to gain a user perspective by examining interactions between family planning clinic staff and their clientele using both objective and subjective research methods. The simulated clients were trained individually and as couples to ask for guidance in choosing family planning methods. Immediately after visiting the clinic, the couples were debriefed about their experiences. Subsequently, family planning staff at four clinics were interviewed to add to the accounts of the simulated clients.

The verbal reports provided by the simulated clients on the information they received in the clinics were subjected to a quantitative analysis of overall content. They were scaled on the basis of accuracy and completeness of the information given as well as on measures of the providers' attitude and bias. The results revealed that the information provided by the family planning clinic staff and their general approach to the simulated clients were strongly related to the client's socioeconomic status. While these quantitative data were informative, our understanding of how the cultural barriers in this society condition relationships is greatly enhanced by the investigators' report of their subjective interactions with the clients.

During the first week of the study we became exasperated with what we perceived at first to be simply a methodological problem. We found it extremely difficult to recruit uneducated lower class (group C) people to work for us, despite the attractive salary and short hours we offered for study participation. Time after time we trained new simulated clients who lost their nerve and then made feeble excuses for failing to visit the clinics. One of our trainers became so fed up that he personally escorted a simulated client-couple to the door of the family planning clinic, only to learn the following day that they had bolted as soon as he was out of sight... Most of the group C clients we recruited did not know the location of a single clinic. They did not understand or believe, although we told them many times, that the clinics exist to provide information and services for people like them, that the staff are paid to answer their questions ... The group C simulated clients would not think of demanding better service because they do not perceive that the clinics are "for them." They expected poor treatment and they got it, yet they were reluctant to criticize. (Schuler 1985: 264–65)

Follow-up interviews with the clinic staff confirmed that they had a low estimation of the intelligence of uneducated clients and sent them away without much information. The hierarchy underlying day-to-day social relations in Nepal's society resulted in the staff talking down to clients and trying to dominate them "for their own good." Correspondingly, the low-caste clients became deferent and submissive. In fact, this deference even interfered with the ability of the researchers to get the simulated clients to articulate their real feelings in the debriefing sessions.

CONTRIBUTIONS OF THE SOCIAL SCIENCES TO THE FIELD OF PUBLIC HEALTH

The Key to all scientific progress lies in the development of new concepts that guide our understanding of the world rather than simply the accumulation of scientific facts (Rubinstein, Laughlin, and McManus 1984). The physical sciences were revolutionized by Newton's discovery of the law of gravity and by Einstein's theory of relativity. Fundamental breakthroughs in the biological sciences came with Darwin's theory of evolution and the discovery of the double helix by Watson and Crick. In the history of economic and social theory there are names such as Malthus, Smith, Marx, and Keynes. Each of these conceptual models generated new knowledge by causing a revolutionary reorganization of pre-existing information as well as by guiding the scientific enterprise into the future. Scientific knowledge that is noteworthy at each stage in its conceptual development may be very useful, as demonstrated by the social and technological developments that follow, but we should always recognize that our present understanding is both conditioned by and limited by the currently accepted conceptual models.

From this perspective we can look at the scientific advancements in public health. A major conceptual breakthrough in our understanding of disease causation came with the Industrial Revolution, which led to the new science of sanitary engineering. Briscoe (1984) identifies three facets of the Industrial Revolution that were the underpinnings of sanitary engineering: first, the unprecedented growth in urban settlements; second, the central tenet of the Industrial Revolution that practical material problems could be solved through the development and application of scientific principles; and third, the political revolutions and unrest that led to an increasing concern with the economic and social conditions of the working class. In this early period, the social reformers who had major influence on public health policy and programs came from the social sciences (Engels), the biological sciences (Virchow), and engineering (Chadwick). The empirical investigations linking abysmal social conditions to disease and death provided sufficient "scientific knowledge" to drive the sanitary reform in Europe in the early nineteenth century even though an organizing scientific theory did not yet exist. As Dubos points out: "What gives special interest to these achievements is that they must be credited to the anti-filth programs organized by boards of health and other municipal bodies that did not believe in contagion, let alone in the germ theory of disease" (Dubos 1959: 149, cited in Tekce 1985).

The development of the germ theory in the latter part of the nineteenth century by Pasteur, Koch, and others provided the critical biological link between environmental conditions and health. The initial inference that there were specific biological agents for many diseases came through critical observations of the interrelationships between human behavior and disease patterns, thus giving birth to the science of epidemiology.[1]

Germ theory and the attendant biological revolution provided the basis for a holistic conceptual framework for health that could take into account social and economic factors, the environment, and individual behavior. However, as scientific knowledge advanced in the twentieth century, disciplinary specialties and subspecialities emerged, not only isolating biomedical scientists from social scientists but even creating barriers to communication among subfields within the respective disciplines. The gap between the biomedical and social scientists was no doubt widened by the Flexner Report in the early part of this century; the report revolutionized medical education, firmly establishing it on a foundation of the biological sciences. Because of the tremendous power of biomedical technology in controlling the highly prevalent communicable diseases, initially through environmental engineering and vaccines and later through the discovery of vitamins and therapeutic interventions, the research agenda in health and disease became synonymous with research in engineering and the biomedical sciences.

Briscoe describes what this meant for the field of sanitary engineering by observing that after several decades of dramatic advances in the late nineteenth and early twentieth century, the scope of the discipline gradually was "reduced to the narrow technical dimensions characteristic of the 'mature' profession" (1984: 239). He draws the interesting parallel that

with this loss of holistic perspective, the discipline has undergone a process akin to the "involution" described by anthropologists in which human cultures, after developing a pattern for responding to an initial challenge, meet all new challenges by ever increasing internal sophistication and differentiation rather than by developing creative and new systemic responses. (Briscoe, citing Geertz 1966: 240)

Broadly speaking, the same judgment could be made for biomedical sciences as they relate to the production of health. While incredible scientific advances have been achieved in the last 50 years, the primary approach to new challenges too often continues to be a search for new and better technologies rather than the study of health problems in all of their dimensions. For example, more and better vaccines are looked to as a solution for a wide array of health problems with major social, economic, ecological, and behavioral determinants including diarrheal diseases, malaria, sexually transmitted diseases, and AIDS.[2]

In the last decade in developed countries there has been a disenchantment with the promises of increasingly sophisticated medical technologies as a solution to the health problems afflicting the population. This is leading to a return to a holistic concept of the determinants of health and disease, as attested by a growing body of research and national policy and position papers by a range of private and government agencies and institutions on these issues (Nightingale 1981). This means, of course, that a research program built around the theme of the health transition is not so much breaking new ground as returning to plow old fields that have lain fallow for many decades. Recent conceptual advances in our understanding of the interrelationships of social conditions and health are a part of this process.

In the field of sanitary engineering, a major conceptual breakthrough in our understanding of the relationships between water and disease came with the work of Bradley, who developed a simple classification that identified the four mechanisms for transmission of all water-related diseases (Bradley and Emurwon 1968). This classification system, given in Table 10.1, provides a concise way of looking at the transmission dynamics of several dozen bacterial, viral, and parasitic diseases asso-

Table 10.1
The Four Mechanisms of Water-Related Disease Transmission and the
Preventive Strategies Appropriate to Each Mechanism

Transmission Mechanism	Preventive Strategy
Waterborne	Improved water quality Prevent casual use of other unimproved sources
Water-washed	Improve water quality Improve water accessibility Improve hygiene
Water-based	Decrease need for water contact Control snail populations Improve quality
Water-related insect vector	Improve surface water management Destroy breeding sites of insects Decrease need to visit breeding sites

Source: Feachem, et al. 1978

ciated with water. More important, it provides a mechanism of linking specific preventive strategies (social interventions) to a multiplicity of water-related diseases through a few basic transmission mechanisms. As Briscoe (1984) observes, this conceptual model has reinvigorated the discipline of sanitary engineering as it relates to health problems in developing countries. It expands the vision of the scientists beyond the issues of technology to ask a range of questions relating to the social, economic, and behavioral problems that may be encountered when attempting to improve water supplies in these settings.[3]

A similar conceptual breakthrough linking biological processes to their social determinants was achieved by Davis and Blake (1956) in their classic model of the proximate determinants of fertility (Table 10.2). Bongaarts (1972) subsequently developed an elegant quantitative model that vastly simplified the problems of measuring the proximate determinants and relating them to overall levels of fertility. This quantitative technique has been applied in fertility surveys worldwide, vastly increasing our objective knowledge about the relative contribution of proximate determinants to different levels of fertility in different societies. In contrast, however, the full potential of the Davis/Blake conceptual model as a framework for elucidating underlying determinants has barely been exploited in developing country settings; thus, our knowledge of the underlying social processes that result in the behaviors mea-

Table 10.2
Intermediate Variables Affecting Fertility

I.	Factors affecting exposure to intercourse		
	A.	Those governing the formation and dissolution of unions in the reproductive period	
		1.	Age of entry into sexual unions
		2.	Permanent celibacy; proportion of women never entering sexual unions
		3.	Amount of reproductive period spent after or between unions
			a. When unions are broken by divorce, separation, or desertion
			b. When unions are broken by death of husband
	B.	Those governing the exposure to intercourse within unions	
		4.	Voluntary abstinence
		5.	Involuntary abstinence (from impotence, illness, and unavoidable but temporary separations)
		6.	Coital frequency (excluding periods of abstinence)
II.	Factors affecting exposure to conception		
		7.	Fecundity or infecundity, as affected by involuntary causes
		8.	Use or nonuse of contraception
			a. By mechanical and chemical means
			b. By other means
		9.	Fecundity or infecundity, as affected by voluntary causes (sterilization, subincision, medical treatment, etc.)
III.	Factors affecting gestation and successful parturition		
		10.	Foetal mortality from involuntary causes
		11.	Foetal mortality from voluntary causes

Source: Davis and Blake 1956.

sured as proximate determinants remains extremely limited for most developing countries (Blake 1983).

Mosley and Chen (1984), following the lead of Davis and Blake, have developed a proximate determinants model of child survival, linking social and economic factors to behavioral mechanisms that result in the biological outcomes of morbidity, growth faltering, and death. Table 10.3 illustrates how a wide range of social and behavioral factors can be related to health outcomes with this model. The insights from this con-

Table 10.3

Intermediate Variables, Biological Indicators of Their Operation on Health, and Some Socioeconomic Determinants

INTERMEDIATE VARIABLES

Physical or biological indicator of health consequences	Some socioeconomic and behavioral factors related to each variable

A. MATERNAL FACTORS

Age
Parity
Interpregnancy interval
  Weight and/or physical development of newborn
  and/or complications of pregnancy and childbirth

Customary age at marriage or first sexual union
Desired family size
Birthspacing
Beliefs about fertility control
Knowledge of methods of contraception and abortion
Accessibility of services
Practice of abstinence
Breast-feeding practices
Use of bottles

B. DIETARY INTAKE (both maternal during pregnancy, and child)

Energy
  Weight at birth (for maternal diet)
  Rate of growth of infant
  Marasmus
Protein
  Kwashiorkor, edema, low serum protein
Vitamins
  Physical signs, e.g., eye disease blindness for
    vitamin A
Minerals
  Anemia
  Goiter, cretinism

Sufficient income to buy food
Food preferences
Method of food preparation
Intrafamilial food distribution
Food taboos
Special dietary practices (restrictions) with pregnancy
  or illness
Breast-feeding, supplement, and weaning practices
Ecological setting
Markets
Food pricing policies
Geographic area of residence (iodine)
Fortification of food

C. ENVIRONMENTAL CONTAMINATION (maternal and infant infection)

Air
  Incidence of respiratory transmitted diseases
    (colds, influenza, pneumonia, diphtheria,
    meningitis, whooping cough, etc.)
  Prevalence of tuberculosis
Food/water/fingers
  Incidence of diarrhea, dysentery, cholera, typhoid
  Prevalence of roundworms
Skin/fomites/soil
  Incidence of skin infection, tetanus (especially
    newborn)
  Prevalence of trachoma, yaws, scabies, lice,
    hookworm
Vectors
  Prevalence of malaria, etc.

Presence of infected persons
Household congestion, indoor fireplaces, ventilation
Water sources, supply, quality, boiling, storage
Food preparation, storage, refrigeration
Use of soap, washing of hands, utensils
Separate kitchen facilities
Bathing and clothes washing practices
Latrine facilities
Sewers
Hygienic practice at childbirth
Geographical area of residence
Vector control programs
Use of screens, netting, insecticides

D. INJURIES

Unintentional injury
  Incidence of physical injuries
  Poisoning
  Prevalence of disabilities due to injury
Intentional injury
  Homicide
  Other violence

Quality of housing, protected fireplaces, safe storage
  for injurious instruments and poisons
Child care practices, protected play areas, etc.

E. DISEASE CONTROL FACTORS

Personal preventive measures
  Incidence of immunizable diseases (diphtheria,
    tetanus, whooping cough; polio, measles,
    tuberculosis)
  Prevalence of malaria, etc.
  Pregnancy complications
Treatments
  Recoveries, disabilities, or deaths with treatments

Beliefs and knowledge about disease causation
Income
Preferences for type of care
Availability and accessibility of preventive and/or
  curative services
Confidence in providers
Cost of prevention or treatment
Use of immunization, prophylactic medicines, e.g.,
  antimalarials, dietary supplements (vitamins, iron)
Antenatal and maternity care
Type of therapy given for each specific condition

Source: Mosley 1989

ceptual approach have stimulated research on organizing data into explanatory models as well as on developing new and improved methodologies to measure the proximate behaviors and relate them to the biological outcomes.

It should be clear from these examples that as we return to a holistic view of the production of health in societies, there will remain a great scope for innovative conceptual models and analytical approaches to social science research. For example, we have little knowledge about the interrelationships between economic development and health, particularly among adults. Also, there are the health systems, both formal and informal, that interact with each other and are jointly used by the population. We need much more understanding of these interactions if new technologies and programs are to be effective and efficient.

MAKING A DIFFERENCE WITH SOCIAL SCIENCE RESEARCH

Can social science research make a difference in the delivery of health care? The answer is unequivocally "yes." We already have the necessary biomedical knowledge and technologies to drive infant mortality rates as low as 10 per 1,000 and life expectancies to upwards of 80 years; thus, it is fair to say that the health differentials we observe between and within national populations are attributable almost entirely to social and economic factors. Most encouraging, the constraints to better health are not intrinsically economic, as illustrated by the fact that many countries and regions with relatively low incomes such as China, Sri Lanka, and the state of Kerala in India enjoy relatively high life expectancies. The question, then, is how social science research can lead to social change.

Before answering this question we must first consider who determines the research agenda. At present the research agenda in developing countries is largely driven by the international donor community—international agencies, bilateral donors, and private foundations—with relatively little support from national governments or indigenous organizations. This is an issue of fundamental importance, since it means the research questions will be largely defined by external agencies to support their institutional objectives rather than by national governments or local institutions, much less by individual scientists working in specific settings.

One may contrast this with the situation in developed countries, taking the United States as an example. As noted earlier, in the now developed world social change was historically driven by individual social reformers, many of whom were scientists working at cross-purposes with government or institutional policies. Today there are a multiplicity of institutions and organizations in the United States engaged in social science and policy research such as the Alan Guttmacher Institute, the Children's Defense Fund, the Urban Institute, the American Cancer Society, the Environmental Defense Fund, the Sierra Club, the American Public Health Association, and dozens of university centers. The work of these institutions is greatly facilitated by the vast array of data generated by local and federal government agencies such as the National Center for Health Statistics. In contrast to all of this, in many developing countries not only are the numbers of social science researchers limited but (this is significant) there are very few autonomous institutions with resources to pursue their independent agendas. Also, in many settings the researchers are constrained by monolithic political systems.

In the international arena we therefore find that most social science research is driven by donor community demand. Consequently, the agenda is largely predefined to support their programmatic objectives. In most cases this means asking a limited number of "objective" questions in support of selective primary health care interventions rather than asking more fundamental questions about the interrelationships of social and economic processes to health conditions. Citing a few examples of programs supported by the Agency for International Development (AID), at the global level we see this focus in the Demographic and Health Surveys (DHS). The Johns Hopkins University under a Child Survival Cooperative Agreement receives support to conduct national sample surveys in selected countries primarily to measure the intermediate outcomes and demographic impact of diarrheal disease control and immunization programs (called Tier II and Tier III program performance indicators). The Primary Health Care Operations Research (PRICOR) project consists in large measure of fine-tuning immunization and oral rehydration service delivery programs. The "missed opportunities" research supported by the World Health Organization (WHO) is limited to examining the health system in terms of its failure to reach children with immunizations. While each of these projects will add incrementally to our knowledge, intellectual breakthroughs are unlikely when the researcher must deliver a predetermined product to the sponsoring agency.

Given these constraints, what can be done—particularly relating to the delivery of health care? Let us look at what is termed "intervention" research. In developing new interventions to strengthen the health service delivery system, the typical approach is to carry out a small-scale pilot project to test its efficacy in a population setting. Historically this research was largely conducted by biomedical scientists focusing on the health impacts of the interventions with little grasp of the social processes involved in their success or failure (Gwatkin, Wilcox, and Wray 1980). In recent years, with the recognition that health interventions are fundamentally social behavioral interventions facilitated by technology, social scientists have become deeply involved in these projects, bringing their analytical and methodological insights into the study design and evaluation.[4] While this step will certainly improve the quality of the product, the question remains whether a pilot project can be successfully translated into a large-scale program that will impact upon health. It turns out that this depends not so much on the results of the projects as on the process of carrying out the research.

In a classic article, Korten (1980) distinguishes two alternative strategies for development programming, the "blueprint" approach and the "learning-process" approach. In the blueprint approach;

researchers are supposed to provide data from pilot projects and other studies which will allow the planners to choose the most cost-effective project design for achieving a given development outcome and to reduce it to a blueprint for implementation. Administrators of the implementing organization are supposed to execute the project faithfully much as a contractor would follow construction blueprints, specifications, and schedules. An evaluation researcher is supposed to measure actual changes in the target population and to report actual versus planned changes to the planners at the end of the project cycle so that the blueprints can be revised. (Korten 1980: 496)

The appeal of the "selective" primary health care approach to the donor community is no doubt in large measure related to the degree to which the technological interventions appear amenable to a blueprint approach. Noteworthy in this approach is that "where the need is for a close integration of knowledge-building, decision-making, and action-taking roles, it sharply differentiates the functions and even the institutional locations of the researcher, the planner, and the administrator" (Korten 1980: 497). It is not surprising that many health intervention programs are falling far short of their objectives because they have failed to achieve a fit between program design, beneficiary need, and the capacities of the assisting organization.[5] Even when they do operate on a large scale, the failure of the project design to take into account the institutional and resource constraints of the recipient country has now led to a new problem (and a new research agenda for social scientists): how to assure financial sustainability (UNICEF 1988).

As an alternative to the blueprint approach, Korten proposes the learning-process approach. In analyzing a number of successful rural development programs in Asia, he observes:

These five programs were not designed and implemented. Rather they emerged out of a learning process in which the villagers and the program personnel shared their knowledge and resources to create a program which achieved a fit between the needs and capacities of the beneficiaries and those of the outsiders who were providing the assistance. Leadership and teamwork, rather than blueprints, were the key elements ... As progress was made in dealing with the problem of fit between beneficiary and program, attention was given either to building a supporting organization around the requirements of the program or adapting the capabilities of an existing organization to fit those requirements. Both program and organization emerged out of a learning process in which research and action were integrally linked. (Korten 1980: 497)

Essential characteristics of a learning organization are that they (1) embrace error; (2) plan with the people; and (3) link knowledge-building with action. Embracing error requires the intellectual integrity to look upon errors and failures to achieve desired outcomes as critical data for making program adjustments to achieve a better fit with beneficiary needs. Planning with the people implies a willingness to accept and use the knowledge, ideas, and resources that the beneficiaries have. This requires close and continuous communication between the implementing organization's members and the community to build on their existing capacity rather than creating a dependence on external resources. In contrast to the blueprint approach where there is sharp differentiation between the roles of researcher, planner, and administrator, linking knowledge with action implies that a learning organization will integrate these functions in a single individual or a close-knit team. This assures the continuous rapid creative adaptation that is necessary to optimize the fit between the program, the organization, and the beneficiaries.

Korten (1980) makes the important observation that in most pilot projects there is indeed a close link between the researcher, the planner, and the administrator. Thus, these projects are typically highly successful in achieving the desired objective. However, at the end of the project the team is disbanded and all that is left is a scientific report that serves as the blueprint for another very different organization, typically a government agency that played no role in the original project. Since the government bureaucracy has none of the characteristics of the project organization, it is not surprising that efforts to replicate the results in a large-scale program fail (Pyle 1982).

The key point is that the learning process must be carried out by, or within the framework of, the organization that will ultimately be responsible for implementing the large-scale program. In this context, Korten (1980) identifies three stages of the learning process. Stage one is learning to be effective. This involves developing a working program model, typically in a village-level learning laboratory. This stage will require a high degree of intellectual input and freedom to experiment and adapt with minimal administration constraints. Here there will be rich opportunities for social scientists, including anthropologists, sociologists, epidemiologists, economists, and others, since this stage will require an in-depth understanding of the social, economic, political, cultural, and ecological dynamics of the community.[6]

Stage two is learning to be efficient. Here activities will have to be standardized and the program design modified to take into account the capabilities of the implementing organization. Traditional operations research projects will be appropriate here; however, there are important roles for social scientists engaged in in-depth studies to understand the dynamics of the organizational structure and to define critical elements in the interaction between the beneficiaries and the provider.

Finally, stage three is learning to expand. Here, again, there will need to be continual refinements of the organizational structure. Research will have to focus on practical ways of measuring organizational performance in terms of input and output variables that are actually related to program impact.

CONCLUSION

It should be clear that social science researchers can be key actors in accelerating the health transition, since health intervention programs are fundamentally social interventions facilitated by technology. In only a few circumstances can technologies be applied involuntarily, such as with mass insecticide application for vector control. There are other areas in public health where social change will be imposed through the political process. This is particularly effective in developed countries with strong governments where there are thousands of laws, regulations, and codes designed to protect the air we breathe, the water we drink, the food we eat, the clothes we wear, the cars we drive, the workplace, the homes we live in, and so forth. There is even control of the information we receive in terms of what can be legitimately advertised. There will always be need for imposed behavior change to protect health, particularly in developing countries, as political systems gain the resources to govern more effectively. At the same time, the vast arenas of human behavior that impact on health will not be subject to explicit government control and regulation. Here, government policies regulating prices, taxes, subsidies, and information, as well as direct investments in services, will implicitly influence health behavior. This is where we need to understand what are the determinants of that behavior, what are its consequences for health, and how intervention programs can improve the situation.

Social scientists are continuing to develop new concepts and tools to understand the social dynamics of societies. One problem, however, is that as the tools and methods become more sophisticated, the presentation of the results often becomes more obscure to the uninitiated. If social scientists are to effectively participate in the process of social change, they must translate their research into products that are not only comprehensible to the consumer but timely as well. In developed countries this is typically done by highly qualified professionals in a wide range of advocacy organizations that are seeking to influence the political process. In developing country settings, these institutions rarely exist; therefore, social scientists will need to develop the tools for rapid data collection and the skills for analyses relevant to action.

Again returning to Korten, he observed that social scientists working in Third World organizations that were effectively building programs through a learning process approach had the following characteristics:

They have sought to demystify the social sciences making it every person's tool, turning both agency personnel and in some instances the villagers themselves into more effective action researchers. They have stressed disciplined observation, guided interviews, and informant panels over formal surveys; timeliness over rigor; oral over written communications; informed interpretation over statistical analysis; narrative over numerical presentation; and attention to the process and intermediate outcomes as a basis for rapid adaptation over detailed assessment of "final" outcomes. Rather than the static profiles provided by typical socioeconomic surveys, they have sought an understanding of the dynamics of the sociotechnical systems that govern village life as a basis for improving predictions of the consequences of any given development intervention. They have sought specific identification of target group members and behavior in terms relevant to program action. (Korten 1980: 501)

Precedents for this approach can be formed in the health field if one is willing to accept that the introduction of family planning technology is a health intervention. A number of national family planning programs, particularly in Asia, were systematically built on a base of social science research gained through a learning-process approach. A classic example is Taiwan.[7] A key characteristic of these programs was the direct link between social science researchers, both national and international, and the program planners and managers. The close involvement of social science researchers with program design, management, implementation, and evaluation resulted in the development of a wide range of new methodologies and analytical approaches that are directly applicable to the strengthening of primary health care programs (Bhatia, Saadah, and Mosley 1989).

The key to effecting institutional and social changes that will lead to health improvements lies not only with the products of social science but also with the research process. Social scientists must bring not only their disciplinary skills but also an interest and commitment to the problem and a willingness to communicate effectively and to listen—not only to their colleagues but to those in other disciplines, as well as in the implementing organizations and the beneficiary communities. To move toward this goal, the international donor community and national agencies in developing countries must recognize that health development is a learning process, and then they must support the development of institutions and scientists who are committed to proceeding on this path.

NOTES

1. John Snow's classic studies on cholera are particularly instructive as case studies combining quantitative and qualitative data. In Snow's "On the Mode of Communication of Cholera" (1855), in addition to providing an extensive quantitative analysis of the problem, he often considered in detail the behavioral characteristics of persons in different social and economic strata to reinforce his theory that cholera is a waterborne disease. For instance, he observed the very high rates among sailors, ballast-heavers, coal porters, and coal-heavers who worked along the river as well as hawkers, tanners, and weavers who lived under crowded, unsanitary conditions. In contrast, he noted that other poor persons such as footmen and manservants who lived in the best part of town with their masters were relatively unaffected. He even made a point about a single case that is worthy of quotation:

There is one remarkable circumstance connected with Dr. Guy's table. One master-brewer died of cholera, being 1 in 160 of the trade; but no brewer's man or brewer's servant is mentioned as having died of this malady, although these men must constitute a very numerous body in London. There must be a few thousand of them. I have, indeed, met with the deaths of two or three of these persons in looking over the returns of some of the most fatal weeks in 1849; but brewers' men seem to have suffered very slightly both in that and the more recent epidemics. The reason of this probably is, that they never drink water, and are therefore exempted from imbibing the cholera poison in that vehicle. (1855: 122–24)

2. The limitations of this "involuted" approach, even in the developed world, are well illustrated in the area of cancer research. In spite of hundreds of millions of dollars invested in Biomedical research on cancer over the last 20 years by the National Institutes of Health, relatively little progress has been made except for a few specific cancers, most notably childhood leukemia. We now appreciate that the major determinants are environmental and behavioral (Nightingale 1981).

3. Among the major investigations building on this conceptual model are two studies: "drawers of Water: Domestic Water Use in East Africa" by White, Bradley, and White (1972) and the multidisciplinary evaluation of water supplies in Lesotho led by Richard Feachem titled "Water, Health, and Development" (1978).

4. A paper presented at a recent interdisciplinary scientific meeting, "Improving Infant Feeding Practices to Prevent Diarrhea and Reduce Its Severity," provides an excellent review of recent experiences and the state of the art in intervention research design (Schroeder, Piwotz, Black, and Kirkwood 1989).

5. UNICEF regularly publishes an Evaluation Newsletter, which provides a timely summary of the organization's health intervention project experiences and openly discusses many problems with achieving its objectives. A case in

point has been the difficulties with the mass campaign approach to immunizations in several sub-Saharan African countries (UNICEF 1989).

6. The project using simulated clients by Schuler, McIntosh, Goldstein, and Pande (1985) could be an example of one "diagnostic" strategy that would be appropriate in this stage of the learning process. What is missing (at least in that published report) is any extended interaction with the providers and the beneficiaries as well as with program managers to get their views on appropriate steps toward solving these problems. Instead, the conclusions and policy recommendations are prescribed by the researchers and senior planners.

7. For Taiwan, see the collection of articles by Cernada (1970). Much of this research has been published in *Studies in Family Planning*, and from time to time the lessons learned have been critically reviewed, most notably by Berelson (1988).

REFERENCES

Berelson, B. 1988. *Berelson on Population.* J. Ross and P. Mauldin, eds. New York: Springer-Verlag.

Bhatia, S., F. Saadah, and W. H. Mosley. 1989. *Analytical Review of the Development of Family Planning Program Strategies, Operations, and Research as a Model for Primary Health Care Programs.* Paper prepared for the International Commission on Health Research for Development, Johns Hopkins University, Baltimore.

Blake, J. 1983. Review of "World Fertility Survey Conference 1980: Record of Proceedings." *Population and Development Review* 9:1:153–56.

Bledsoe, C. 1989. *Unravelling the Trickle-Down Model within Households: Foster Children and the Phenomenon of Scrounging.* Paper presented at the Rockefeller Foundation Exploratory Health Transition Program, Workshop No. 2, "Methods for Studying Health Transition Processes," London.

Bongaarts, J. 1978. A Framework for Analyzing the Proximate Determinants of Fertility. *Population and Development Review* 4:1:105–32.

Bradley, D. J. 1977. Health Aspects of Water Supplies in Tropical Countries. In *Water, Wastes and Health in Hot Climates.* R. G. Feachem, M. McGarry, and D. D. Mara, eds. London: Wiley.

Bradley, D. J., and P. Emurwon. 1968. Predicting the Epidemiological Effects of Changing Water Sources. *East African Medical Journal* 45:284–91.

Briscoe, J. 1984. Technology and Child Survival: The Example of Sanitary Engineering. In *Child Survival: Strategies for Research.* W. H. Mosley and L. C. Chen, eds. A supplement to Vol. 10 of *Population and Development Review.* New York: Population Council.

Cebu Study Team. 1991. Underlying and Proximate Determinants of Child Health: The 1988 Cebu Longitudinal Health and Nutrition Study. *American Journal of Epidemiology* 133:2:185–201.

Cernada, G. P. ed. 1970. *Taiwan Family Planning Reader: How A Program Works.* Taichung, Taiwan: Chinese Center for International Training in Family Planning, and New York: Population Council.

Davis, D., and J. Blake. 1956. Social Structure and Fertility: An Analytic Framework. *Economic Development and Cultural Change* 4:211–35.

Dubos, R. 1959. *Mirage of Health: Utopias, Progress, and Biological Change.* Republished in 1979. New York: Harper and Row.

Feachem, R., E. Burns, S. Cavincross, A. Cronin, P. Cross, D. Curtis, M. K. Khan, D. Lamb, and H. Southall. 1978. *Water, Health, and Development: An Interdisciplinary Evaluation.* London: Tri-med Books Ltd.

Geertz, G. C. 1966. *Agricultural Involution: The Process of Ecological Change in Indonesia.* Berkeley: University of California Press.

Gwatkin, D. R., J. R. Wilcox, and J. D. Wray. 1980. *Can Health and Nutrition Intervention Make a Difference?* Washington, D.C.: Overseas Development Council.

Korten, D. C. 1980. Community Organization and Rural Development: A Learning Process Approach. *Public Administration Review* (September/October): 480–511.

Mosley, W. H. 1989. Interactions of Technologies with the Household Production of Health. In *Toward More Efficacy in Child Survival Strategies: Understanding the Social and Private Constraints and Responsibilities.* I. Sirageldin, W. H. Mosley, R. Levine, V. Schwoebel, and K. Horiuchi, eds. Baltimore, Md.: Johns Hopkins University.

Mosley, W. H., and L. C. Chen. 1984. An Analytical Framework for the Study of Child Survival in Developing Countries. In *Child Survival: Strategies for Research.* W. H. Mosley and L. C. Chen, eds. A supplement to Vol. 10 of *Population and Development Review.* New York: Population Council.

Nightingale, E. 1981. *Prospects for Reducing Mortality in Developed Countries by Changes in Day-to-Day Behavior.* Vol. 2, International Population Conference Proceedings, Manila, 1981. Liege, Belgium: International Union for the Scientific Study of Population. IUSSP.

Pyle, D. F. 1982. *From Project to Program: Structural Constraints Associated with Expansion.* National Association of Schools of Public Affairs and Administration Working Paper No. 3 in cooperation with USAID, Office of Science and Technology. Washington D.C.: Agency for International Development, U.S. Department of State.

Rubinstein, R. A. 1984. Epidemiology and Anthropology: Notes on Science and Scientism. *Communication and Cognition* 17:2/3:163–85.

Rubinstein, R. A., C. D. Laughlin, and J. McManus. 1984. *Science as Cognitive Process: Toward an Empirical Philosophy of Science.* Philadelphia: University of Pennsylvania Press.

Schroeder, D. G., E. G. Piwotz, R. E. Black, and B. R. Kirkwood. 1989. *Improving Infant Feeding Practices to Prevent Diarrhea and Reduce Its Severity: Intervention Research Priorities and Methodological Considerations.* Occasional Paper No. 8, Institute for International Programs. Baltimore, M.D.: Johns Hopkins University.

Schuler, S. R., E. N. McIntosh, M. C. Goldstein, B. R. Pande. 1985. Barriers to Effective Family Planning in Nepal. *Studies in Family Planning* 16 (September/October):5.

Snow, J. 1855. On the Communication of Cholera. In *Snow on Cholera: A Reprint of Two Papers.* London: John Churchill, 1936.

Tekce, B. 1985. Determinants of Child Survival: Comments on a New Perspective. In *Population Factors in Development Planning in the Middle East*. F. C. Shorter and H. Zurayk, eds. New York: Population Council.

UNICEF. 1988. *Problems and Priorities regarding Recurrent Costs, A UNICEF Policy Review*. New York: UNICEF.

——. 1989. *Evaluation Newsletter*, No. 8, May.

White, G. F., D. J. Bradley, and A. U. White. 1972. *Drawers of Water: Domestic Water Use in East Africa*. Chicago: University of Chicago Press.

The Health Transition and Social Science Research: A Summary of Workshop Proceedings

LINCOLN C. CHEN

As indicated in the introduction, the workshop on which this book is based was the third of a series on the health transition sponsored by the Rockefeller Foundation. The first, in Canberra, addressed the question: What is the health transition? The second, in London, asked: How does one go about studying the health transition? This third and final workshop posed the challenge: How does social science research relate to health policy and action?

The workshop was organized into three parts. On the first day, we reviewed the fields of health behavior, politics, economics, and health care systems. A number of case studies were discussed on the second day. Additional attractions were the first day's dinner speech by William Foege on the necessity of social research for social action, and the spontaneous and candid after-dinner exchange on the second day, which centered on issues of North-South relations. Also noteworthy was the reaffirmation of the fundamental importance of research capacity building within developing countries.

The highlight of the event, in my opinion, was the concluding sessions on the third day. The morning panelists succeeded in synthesizing the earlier sessions by integrating research areas and specific problems, basing their assessments on their own rich and diverse experiences. Just before the final session, smaller working groups formulated specific recommendations directed to three audiences: national governments, international agencies, and development (nongovernmental) action projects.

This summary is divided into four parts. It begins with a preliminary review of several unresolved challenges raised by participants, then addresses, in turn, three basic questions: (1) Is the health transition concept useful? (2) What are the linkages between social research and social action? (3) How can an evolving health transition program make a difference?

UNRESOLVED CHALLENGES

Nirmala Murthy posed the first challenge when she observed, "Patients need doctors, but who needs a social scientist?" The question is simple; yet it effectively sums up the major challenge to which the health transition program must respond. One possible response is that as long as medical practice deals with the care of individuals, the social sciences are needed by populations, communities, and other groups. For many, if not most, of the major questions about determinants of health cannot be addressed by individually oriented medicine. Health equity, for example, involves the distribution of resources among individuals in populations. Health promotion and prevention, as noted in this workshop, are very much socially conditioned phenomena. Even most health care policies and programs depend upon population-based approaches.

A second challenge came from Achola Pala Okeyo: "How does social science make a difference in the everyday lives of people living in a community?" Unlike the natural sciences, the social sciences do not produce "magic bullet" technologies that immediately solve practical problems. Rather, as David Mechanic reminded us, the social sciences deal with extremely complex behavioral and social systems that can change only slowly. While resistant to change, these human systems are also extremely powerful and undoubtedly have profound health implications.

On the last night, Elias Sevilla-Casas diplomatically offered the third challenge. Recounting the process by which a major international funding agency was asked to leave Colombian universities in 1975, he concluded with the following central concern: Given an understanding of changing contexts and a willingness to learn from experience, how can a new program, such as the health transition program, create a new relationship with a given agency? The careful crafting of collaboration and communication patterns, together with the development of shared values and commitment, is required.

SIGNIFICANCE AND USEFULNESS OF THE HEALTH TRANSITION CONCEPT

The timeliness and significance of the health transition concept was reaffirmed by all participants. David Mechanic argued for the importance of "psychological modernity" in influencing health attitudes, behavior, and outcomes in industrialized countries. Stephen Weiss reviewed the contribution of multidisciplinary behavioral approaches to health promotion. Arthur Kleinman argued that health behavior is a powerful mediator of health outcomes and that research is needed to document the prevalence of neglected behavioral pathologies, for example, alcohol and drug abuse, mental illness, and other disabling conditions.

In the discussions, Bonnie Stanton and Claudio Lanata reminded us of the importance of household health behavior. The violence and neglect that are so pervasive in industrialized countries, and that are also being recognized in some developing countries (e.g., child neglect in Bangladesh and Peru), are examples of this. It was argued, moreover, that a behavioral focus should not be limited to populations at risk for illness. The attitudes and behaviors of those who control resources (policymakers, academics, donors) also have important health consequences.

In the session on political economy, Michael Reich examined the concept of political commitment and challenged us to reflect upon the fact that some benefit and others suffer from any given health policy. The significance of political and social processes in shaping health policies was vividly illustrated by Daniel Fox's review of AIDS interventions in three industrialized countries, where differing contexts have resulted in varying responses to the epidemic. James Rule noted that the health field, unlike others, has traditionally been cloaked in harmony. After all, preventing and curing illness is a value shared by all! Yet this apparent harmony may also mask a reluctance to confront the conflictual aspects of health, which reflect the distribution of power and resources in society.

A missing link, Nancy Birdsall reminded us, is the absence of scientific work in health economics. Whatever else may be considered important in health, the reality is that in most societies, decisions about the allocation of resources are made by political leaders, who are guided by economic considerations. More research and communication between economists and health scientists are needed.

Dr. Kiwara noted that many developing countries refuse to accept the present reality of having to cope with daunting health threats with far more limited economic resources than industrialized countries possess. He argued that international indebtedness and slow economic growth in developing countries, due in part to an unjust international economic system, powerfully constrain health advances in many parts of the world.

Policies and programs in the health sector are the most direct response to preventable illness and premature death, and information and participation are central to the success of health interventions. A report of an innovative project designed to combat diarrheal disease in Peru, presented by Guillermo Lopez de Romana, illustrated the importance of information, evaluation, and mothers' participation in efforts to implement a dietary management program. The involvement of health workers was shown to be crucial to the success of a survey of immunization coverage in a presentation by Claudio Lanata.

Donald Sawyer and Diana Sawyer examined the resurgence of malaria in the Amazon region, noting that the social sciences are playing an important role in advancing the understanding of disease ecology and transmission that is essential for disease control. Burton Singer, in commenting on the malaria case, noted that high-technology approaches have all too often been inappropriately transferred from industrialized to developing countries. Mass insecticide spraying to combat the malaria vector and chemoprophylaxis directed against the parasite have clearly failed to control the disease. Social science research is needed to develop and promote strategies that are both medically effective and ecologically sound.

Often, the significance of social science research for the health transition was debated. The discussion focused on the search for a definition of social research in health and the identification of a research agenda. Some of the comments even implied that the concept of health itself should be redefined. The argument here is that enormous growth in health promotion activities and changes in health behavior in industrialized countries have altered the traditional concept of health as a product of curative medical practice. Illness is no longer visualized as a haphazard event, but rather as a consequence of lifestyle. In developing countries health has become inextricably linked to overall development, perceived as both determinant and outcome of the pattern and direction of socioeconomic change. *Health and development,* not just medicine, is emerging as an integrated and viable concept that is relevant to both industrialized and developing countries.

Research itself was also redefined, albeit inconclusively, in the course of the workshop discussions. W. Henry Mosley advanced the proposition that social science research was not simply the familiar hypothesis formulation and testing. Rather, he argued, research includes action. Social research, in Mosley's view, includes the active participation of researchers in intervention—taking risks, dealing with mistakes and errors, and learning from doing.

Yet another challenge was posed in the question: Who sets the research agenda? Academics? Policymakers? Donors? Consensus did not emerge from the debate on this issue. What was clear, however, was that the customary notion of academics being supported by donors to produce research for use by policymakers was naive and simplistic. Indeed, the issue of agenda-setting emerged as central to our next major theme.

SOCIAL RESEARCH AND SOCIAL ACTION

Examining the linkages between social science research and social action requires that the concept of research be more precisely defined. Research can refer to a product or to the process of generating that product. Kenneth Prewitt, for example, challenged the participants to identify key research findings, or products, that could make a health difference. Other participants, in contrast, focused on the processes involved in research production and use. The product versus process debate was not resolved, but there was agreement that the participation of all relevant actors was essential to both.

In moving research into the domain of public discourse and translating research results into public policy, a major challenge (from a scientist's viewpoint) is how to generate demand for research findings from policymakers. Our understanding of this process is minimal. W. Henry Mosley observed that policymakers have answers for the problems they face; they are not looking for questions or hypotheses. Claudio Lanata recounted his frustration in dealings with health policymakers in Peru.

One simple strategy for dealing with this might be to involve policymakers in the formulation of the research agenda. However, Richard Cash argued that this could lead to the subordination of research plans to political and bureaucratic goals, thereby compromising independence, creativity, and productivity.

One of the most valuable roles the social sciences can play, it was pointed out, is that of critic: raising questions, challenging established authority, and ensuring openness in assessing government performance. Nowhere is this role more poignantly visible than in the recent decimation of the intellectual community in China, where social criticism has provoked such violent responses from authoritarian rule.

Two general theories specifying the relationship of research to action were succinctly presented by Michael Reich. In the first, a particular research product is viewed as directly linked to a specific action decision. For an example of this direct linkage, we may look to the consistently successful use private business has made of social science. Demographic studies identify market segments, economic research pinpoints effective demand, and marketing departments invest in mass media campaigns in the hope of influencing consumer attitudes and behavior. The success of the tobacco industry in propagating smoking, first in industrialized countries, and now, increasingly, in the developing world, reveals the power of social science research in the services of business interests. In fact, there emerged from the discussion a call for the application of social sciences to health promotion as a public good, a way of counterbalancing its use for purely commercial purposes. The question may be less whether social science is useful than how to use this clearly effective tool to achieve social goals.

The second theory posits an indirect relation of research to action, in which movement from the former to the latter is mediated by some intervening factor. For David Mechanic, this mediating influence was "social climate," or "a culture of ideas, attitudes, and activities," which shapes the transformation of research results into pragmatic form. On another level, W. Henry Mosley showed us that certain types of intermediary organizations, themselves neither purely research- nor exclusively policy-oriented, can play a similar mediating role.

In the United States, we can point to certain socially conscious advocacy groups—the Sierra Club, the American Cancer Society, the Natural Resource Defense Fund—that have assumed responsibility for mobilizing research results and other information in the public service. Allan Brandt's exposition of the history of tobacco policy in the United States vividly underscores the powerful role of the American Cancer Society in forcing escalation of the exercise of public policy from simple letters to medical journals to a three-hour television show that beamed the Surgeon General himself into American homes.

Does this U.S. model of intermediary organizations have parallels in diverse developing countries? The United States is a pluralistic society with large private sectors, commercial and nonprofit. Institutional forms in much of the developing world, in contrast, are young and fragile. In many countries, recent independence from colonialism has understandably resulted in efforts to strengthen national governments in newly sovereign states. The public sector controlled by the nation state dominates the institutional landscape.

Some exceptions to this pattern exist, and they should be noted. India, for example, has many scientifically based advocacy groups—the Voluntary Health Association of India, the Nutrition Foundation of India, the Center for Science and the Environment. There was a suggestion from Dr. Kiwara that perhaps "inappropriate" exports from industrialized to developing countries (e.g., high-technology disease control strategies) should be abandoned in favor of the transfer of socially oriented scientific advocacy groups. Indeed, it was noted that several American organizations based in Washington, D.C., are providing methodological training for their counterparts in developing countries. These include the Children's Defense Fund and many environmental lobby groups.

A third intervening factor is people—leaders and nonleaders alike. Elias Sevilla-Casas noted that the University of the Andes has a virtually direct channel into the Ministry of Finance in Colombia, due to the movement of people between the university and the government. In Nigeria, contemporary leadership for primary health care is coming from a minister, Dr. Ransome-Kuti, who previously was a professor of pediatrics. During his university tenure, Dr. Ransome-Kuti undertook an experimental community-based health care program. The lessons learned were implemented not through journal articles but through the leadership of an engaged and committed scientist who moved from an academic setting into government.

It was pointed out, however, that people who are not in leadership positions also have an important role to play. Gelia Castillo urged us to focus on the young. In contrast to established scientists, postdoctoral fellows, for example, are less indoctrinated, more willing to go to rural areas, more able to take risks and tolerate mistakes, and less worried about tarnishing their reputations. Young scholars are more likely to listen to people who suffer from, or are at high risk for, poor health. They have a better chance of generating new and creative ideas.

The importance of an enabling environment to facilitate both types of research-to-action linkages was also discussed. The *legitimization* of the social sciences as an appropriate tool for addressing health problems was seen as possibly the most important enabling factor. Neither the powerful medical profession nor social scientists themselves presently view health as suitable subject matter for social research. But whatever the intervening factor, in the linkage process we must attract outstanding social scientists to health research, change perceptions of the roles and responsibilities of the various sciences, and provide peer support and professional recognition for social scientists as an incentive to become involved.

The discussion of social research and social action ended with a penetrating observation by Nirmala Murthy, who noted that fundamentally social scientists and policymakers belong to two distinct cultures. Murthy argued that we cannot assume that training, skill development, and research dissemination will improve research-action linkages between these two cultures. Rather, she proposed that the slow development of shared perceptions and a recognition of the value of each culture's respective role will help the two groups to understand how to use each other more effectively. Murthy recounted her own experience as part of a team of social scientists and health policymakers charged with solving health and population problems in backward states of India, and how this led to mutual learning and respect. These lessons are far more useful than what can be gleaned from a textbook or a course at Harvard.

THE HEALTH TRANSITION PROGRAM

How can a health transition program make a difference? Regrettably but perhaps not unexpectedly, a blueprint did not emerge from the discussions. Rather, some general guidelines for the development of such a program were offered by the workshop participants.

First, a health transition program must struggle to improve the *linkages between research and action.* Either one alone is unproductive, Without a clear link to action, research may wander off into irrelevance. While basic enquiry of course has its place, it is not appropriate for a health transition program. Similarly, action or advocacy uninformed by research can be effective. In this case, however, a pure action approach would simply duplicate the massive investments now being made by national governments and bilateral and multilateral agencies. The situation is too urgent to miss the chance to build capacity, knowledge, and linkages, thereby furthering the application of existing knowledge and creating new knowledge for health advancement.

A second guideline highlights the importance of program *focus and coherence.* Three days of discussions have produced a clear conceptual map of the many directions that might be pursued. However, a program with finite resources must, at least at the outset, be more focused—in terms of the population to be served, the scientists to be involved, the types of problems to be addressed, and the research areas to be targeted. Coherence is critical for a program in the early phases of development, especially where that program, given its inherently interdisciplinary nature, runs the risk of diffusion.

There was nearly unanimous agreement that a *networking* strategy should be attempted in the health transition program. We may look to the renowned International Clinical Epidemiology Network (INCLEN) for an example of a successful network model. Networks can be fashioned in many ways. In the case of the health transition program, the network should foster exchange, nurture research capacity (especially in developing countries), and promote the development of shared values and common purpose among its members. But these questions remain: How should the network promote the collection and analysis of data and the dissemination of research products? How can the network help to increase the pool of social scientists interested in health research? Can partnerships be nurtured—not to pursue the unreachable goal of total equality of skills and resources among members, but to achieve mutual respect? How might the network improve access to information and the scientific literature for those cut off from the flow of data and ideas? Will the network approach encourage a more appropriate transfer of lessons from one setting to another? How should the network ensure the members derive professional satisfaction, as well as personal enjoyment, from participation?

Consistent with the network concept is the notion of timely and adequate *communications among donors.* Gelia Castillo noted that programs similar to the proposed health transition program are currently being supported by a number of different funding agencies. Examples include the Social and Economic Research Group of the WHO Tropical Disease

Program, the WHO Intersectoral Action for Health Program, the International Health Policy Program, and the health programs of the International Development Research Centre (IDRC) in Canada. The aim here is not to bring about "donor coordination," an often invoked but rarely implemented concept, but rather to encourage the sharing of information, the development of joint activities, and the focusing of attention on the needs addressed by this program. Better donor communication is essential to avoid overtaxing social scientists, especially in developing countries where they are few in number and are deluged with research opportunities.

A final guideline to be considered in developing the program is *time*. The workshop participants concurred that a health transition initiative does not fit the model of a two-year project funded by a government agency. Achieving the aims of the program—the building of capacity; the generation, completion and dissemination of research; the construction of linkages between policy and action—will require at least a decade of work. The aspirations of the health transition program—conducting research, changing attitudes, enhancing capabilities—are too ambitious for a project-model approach. Substantial time and patience are required.

At a more concrete level, these guidelines might be implemented as follows: Select a few key participants, develop a critical mass at a few centers within an international network, acquire some program momentum, and maintain a flexible, adaptive, and experimental posture. Include individuals with different backgrounds, because this program needs range and diversity. Introduce focus through regular topical, problem-oriented, or geographically oriented workshops, perhaps at quarterly or semiannual intervals. These gatherings could sequentially address the many unanswered questions posed in this workshop. Bring practitioners and policymakers together with a few scientists (the reverse of this workshop's composition) to talk about links between research and action. Have a workshop on malaria control in the Amazon and include health planners, researchers, health care providers, and leaders from the affected communities. Construct a network to address the question of how the linkage between women's education and family health can be exploited in policy and programs. Through such activities, introduce some element of forward motion and progress, even as the longer-term agenda of capacity building is being pursued. A journal and a newsletter would be useful in keeping network members and other interested parties informed and involved.

The success of the program may revolve more around the engagement of young people than the production of research. The true test may be the number and quality of junior scholars who are attracted to this enterprise, as this generation will emerge as the leaders of the "health for all" movement—not by the year 2000 but certainly by 2025.

The performance of the health transition program should also be evaluated. The evaluation should include not only self-assessment by network members and the funding agencies, but also input from external participants. No formal evaluation, however, will replace the need for faith. There are no cost-effectiveness studies to conclusively prove that a health transition program should be undertaken or that it will generate high health impact at low cost. Rather, the participants will need to trust that what they are engaged in is worthwhile and that it can indeed make a difference in people's everyday lives.

Finally, as exciting as it has been, this workshop, represents only one step in a journey. We are eager to begin. In the meantime, perhaps I can respond to Kenneth Prewitt's request for alternative names for the program of activities we hope to undertake. The term "health transition" was coined by Jack and Pat Caldwell, intellectual pioneers in this field. Some consider the term too neutral or static. But other titles seem too nondescript: "Accelerating the Health Transition," or "Social Research and Action for Health," or "Health and Public Policy." Perhaps, as Elias Sevilla-Casas implied, a most appropriate title would be this: "A Health Transition for All!"

Index

About the Editors and Contributors

LINCOLN C. CHEN is Taro Takemi Professor of International Health, Director of International Health Programs, and Director of the Center for Population and Development Studies at Harvard University. He has published more than 100 articles on international health.

ARTHUR KLEINMAN is Chair of the Department of Social Medicine, Professor of Medical Anthropology, and Professor of Psychiatry at Harvard University. He is the author of *The Illness Narratives* (1988), *Social Origins of Distress and Disease* (1986), and *Advances in Mood Disorders* (with J. Becker, 1990). His works in progress include *Health and Social Change in International Perspective* and *Pain as Human Experience: An Anthropological Perspective*.

NORMA C. WARE is Instructor in Social Medicine at Harvard Medical School. Previously Associate Dean of Radcliffe College, she specializes in medical anthropology and cross-cultural psychiatry.

NANCY BIRDSALL, The World Bank, Washington, D.C.

ROBERT E. BLACK, The Johns Hopkins University

ALLAN M. BRANDT, University of North Carolina

NICHOLAS A. CHRISTAKIS, University of Pennsylvania

HILARY M. CREED, Instituto de Investigacion Nutricional, Lima, Peru

SALLY E. FINDLEY, Columbia University

DANIEL M. FOX, Milbank Memorial Fund

MARY FUKUMOTO, Instituto de Investigacion Nutricional, Lima, Peru

HILDA GONZALES, Instituto de Investigacion Nutricional, Lima, Peru

PRAKASH C. GUPTA, Tata Institute of Fundamental Research, Bombay, India

ENRIQUE R. JACOBY, Instituto de Investigacion Nutricional, Lima, Peru

CLAUDIO F. LANATA, Instituto de Investigacion Nutricional, Lima, Peru

SOFIA S. MADRID, Instituto de Investigacion Nutricional, Lima, Peru

DAVID MECHANIC, Rutgers University

W. HENRY MOSLEY, The Johns Hopkins University

CARLA MAKHLOUF OBERMEYER, Harvard University

GUILLERMO LOPEZ DE ROMANA, Instituto de Investigacion Nutricional, Lima, Peru

DIANA O. SAWYER, Yale University

DONALD R. SAWYER, Instituto Sociedade, Populacao, e Natureza, Brasilia, Brazil

ELIAS SEVILLA-CASAS, Universidad del Valle, Cali, Colombia

GEORGE STROH, JR., Centers for Disease Control, Atlanta, Georgia

STEPHEN M. WEISS, National Institutes of Health

BARBARA O. DE ZALDUONDO, The Johns Hopkins University